ROAD TO RECOVERY

ROAD TO RECOVERY
New Techniques for Healing

Chronic Fatigue Syndrome

Fibromyalgia

Gulf War Syndrome

Rheumatoid Arthritis

Depression

Chronic Yeast Infection

Obesity

Alcoholism

Celiac Disease

Mycoplasma

Heavy Metal Toxicity / Poisoning

Chronic Viral Infections

With Spiritual Insights
    for the Chronically Ill

Marc Herlands, J.D.

RECOVERY PRESS
San Diego, California

ISBN-13: 9781481916912 (Marc Herlands)
ISBN-10: 1481916912

Marc Herlands
Recovery Press
P.O. Box 231746
Encinitas, CA 92023-1746
U.S.A.

A Very Special Thanks to
Paul Lloyd Warner - Project Manager:
Book Design and Typesetting

VISIT OUR WEBSITE AT:
www.RoadToRecoveryBook.com
for additional books, e-books and products

Remedies for:

Chronic Fatigue Syndrome
Fibromyalgia
Gulf War Syndrome
Rheumatoid Arthritis
Depression
Chronic Yeast Infection
Obesity
Alcoholism
Celiac Disease
Mycoplasma
Heavy Metal Toxicity / Poisoning
Chronic Viral Infections
With Spiritual Insights
         for the Chronically Ill

DEDICATIONS
To My Wife and My Other Angels

To my dearest wife, **Louise L. Herlands,** affectionately known to me as "*Louie*," or "*Lou*," the love of my life for 30 years, who never gave up on me, and always encouraged me on my "Road to Recovery." *God Bless You and Your Memory.*

And to all my other angels, including my friends, family, doctors, dentists, healthcare practitioners and supporters, who gave me their unyielding love and understanding on my long "Road to Recovery."

I wish to acknowledge all of you, and thank you, with my life and my love.

My Very Special Thanks To –
Dr. Gary Shima, MD
Health and Longevity Institute
1529 Grand Avenue, Suite B
San Marcos, CA 92078

Ms. Roxanne Watson, CHT

Living Water Rejuvenation Center

5670 El Camino Real

Carlsbad, CA 92008

www.LivingWaterRejuvenation.com

and

Ms. Cathy Brady, JD, LL.M.

Dr. Mark Drucker, MD

Ms. Svetlana Elbert, BS

Dr. Hal Huggins, DDS

Dr. Ronald Lesko, DO

Dr. William Kellas, PhD

Dr. Javier Morales, DDS

Dr. Garth Nicolson, PhD

Mr. Mark J. Olsen, AF

Dr. R. Paul St. Amand, MD

Mr. Dennis Schiller, BA

Ms. Shirley Smith, AS

Mr. William Timmons, ND

All of whom played a direct and very important part in saving my life since 1991.

To My Group
And Others

You may notice that I have published this book with large print, margins and spaces between paragraphs. I did these things on purpose, because I am writing to a group of people --- a group of which I am *proud* to be a life-long *member* --- who needs to take extensive notes about what we have just read.

We need to write the questions *immediately* as they come to mind, because we forget what we were thinking about.

I have used simple language and sentence structure because my group of people has major difficulties reading, comprehending and remembering what we have just read.

Those people who are members of my group know why I did this and appreciate my efforts.

Those who have *empathy* for our problems, our doctors, medical advisors, healers, caregivers, co-workers, bosses, friends and family will understand as well.

Those who do not really know us, do not really understand our challenges. So, I have tried to explain why I have chosen to write my book in this manner.

It was written for members of my group who are cognitively impaired. It was not written for those who are cognitively normal. It was written to give hope and information to those who are not able to think clearly. It was not written for those who are able to function at a normal level of thinking.

If you find yourself thinking this book is way too simple, and so you are thinking about discarding the information contained herein, please consider that my IQ was measured to be in the top 2% of the population, and I have earned a law degree and a master's degree in tax law.

It is not that I am unintelligent. It is that I am writing this book for a specific audience, most of whom have a lot of mental challenges.

If you're one of the lucky ones, meaning - you are *not* a member of *my* group - count yourself very lucky in deed.

The members of my group have it tough, physically, mentally, emotionally and financially.

It is for them I have written this book.

It is for them my heart bleeds.

Best wishes,
Marc Herlands
BA (economics), JD (business), LL.M. (tax)

February, 2013

Disclaimer

Dear Reader: The information provided in this book is *for informational purposes only*. It is *not* to be construed as *medical advice* or *medical care*, and the information herein is *not* a replacement for professional medical advice or care given by licensed physicians or trained medical personnel. The author and publisher do *not* directly or indirectly *practice* medicine. Nor do they dispense medical advice, care, diagnosis, treatment or any other medical service. *Dear Patient*: *Always* seek the advice of your physician or other qualified healthcare provider whenever you experience symptoms or health problems, or before starting any new medical treatment. Please note that the author and publisher are *not* responsible for any inaccuracies, omissions or editorial errors in this book; nor for any consequences resulting from the information provided herein. *Dear Physician*: It is always *your* responsibility to evaluate the information provided herein and the results from the information provided. *Dear Health Care Professional*: You should always exercise your professional judgment when evaluating any information provided herein. We *encourage* you to confirm from other sources that the information provided herein is accurate in all respects *before* undertaking any treatment protocol or any other action which may be based upon the information presented herein.

Table of Contents

Preface

"Road to Recovery – New Techniques for Healing Chronic Fatigue Syndrome, Fibromyalgia, Gulf War Syndrome, Rheumatoid Arthritis, Depression, Chronic Yeast Infection, Obesity, Alcoholism, Celiac Disease, with Spiritual Insights for the Chronically Ill" is the autobiography of Marc Herlands, a young Jewish attorney, who at the age of 26, had his career and personal life totally ruined by chronic exhaustion and terrible emotional problems, which later became known as the Chronic Fatigue Syndrome (CFS), and what he had to do during the next 38 years to totally recover.

His CFS came upon him suddenly in 1974 without apparent cause, and left him unable to practice his profession at the highest levels while he was in his first year of practicing law in Beachwood, Ohio, a suburb of Cleveland.

At the age of 39, in 1989, while he was living in San Diego with his beloved wife, Louise, his life became unbearable. He started to suffer severe pain throughout his body, but especially in his legs (Fibromyalgia). That illness came upon him suddenly, like CFS, without any apparent cause as well.

In 1991, at the age of 43, Marc was so exhausted that he was sleeping 20 hours per day. Ironically, he had to take barbiturates to keep himself asleep because the pain in his legs was so great it woke him up every two hours. Sadly, he was more tired when he awoke in the morning than when he went to bed at night.

In 1991, after 17 years of chronic exhaustion and 4 years of severe pain, suicide became a planned and attractive option.

But, at the end of 1991, at the age of 43, Marc's luck changed for the better. With his wife and a friend from law school, he found Dr. Morales, a dentist in Mexico, Dr. Gary J. Shima, M.D. in Encinitas, and a few other medical practitioners in California who discovered many of the underlying causes of his illnesses, and then began some unconventional treatments which started to relieve a lot of his CFS, Fibromyalgia and depression over the next nine years. But not all.

They found that Marc suffered from the **toxic effects** of excessive amounts of **heavy metals**, such as *lead, mercury, nickel, vanadium and cadmium*, which had accumulated in his body.

He also had a **dysfunctional immune system** and **chronic viral and bacterial infections**. The sum of these parts was the beginning of a theory about why Marc had contracted CFS, Fibromyalgia and depression, and how to remedy those illnesses.

A few years later, Dr. Gary J. Shima, now of San Marcos, California, found that Marc suffered from **yeast and fungus overgrowth** and **Leaky Gut Syndrome**.

Each of those illnesses was a significant cause of his **severe obesity, confusion, depression and internally produced alcoholism.**

Later, another extremely important part of his story came to light. He was diagnosed with having **celiac disease.** That disease (1) prevented him from fully absorbing vitamins and nutrients, (2) stunted his growth, (3) prevented the elimination of toxic heavy metals from his body, (4) created impacted bowel syndrome, and (5) created constant fatigue and pain.

Another important factor in Marc's universe of illnesses was the discovery of his being infected with **mycoplasma fermentans incognitas.**

Dr. Garth Nicolson, Ph.D., a clinical researcher, has testified before the U.S. Congress that the above mycoplasma is the primary cause of the **Gulf War Syndrome.** It is a highly dangerous, contagious debilitating bug that was created as a

Biological Weapon of Mass Destruction by the U.S. government. As such, it is not lethal but totally draining and emotionally destructive. Luckily, Marc has been able to rid himself of that horrible pathogen twice.

Another piece of Marc's medical puzzle was added when he was diagnosed with a **neurological disorder** which caused him to be extremely fatigued, suffer chronic pain and develop hypersensitivities to light, sound and odors.

Luckily, Marc responded well to medicines such as Neurotin (gabapentin), which reduced his fatigue and pain, and Lamictal, which reduced his hypersensitivities light, sound and odors.

By 2002, at the age of 54, after almost ten years of treatments and remedies, which included the use of *medicines, antibiotics, oxygen, transfer factor, vitamins, minerals, herbs, amino acids, enzymes, essential fatty acids, chelation, colonics, acupuncture, chiropractic, lymph massage, diet changes, yoga, meditation, and removing the silver/mercury fillings from his teeth,* Marc's health greatly improved. But not enough. He was still tired and mentally challenged. His short term memory and his vitality were still very limited.

But, by 2012, the Chronic Fatigue Syndrome's exhaustion, the Fibromyalgia's pain, the depression and brain fog have gone, and he has recovered.

Beginning in 1974, at the age of 26, and for the next 38 years, Marc consulted with over 100 doctors, healers, and health care providers trying to (1) discover the causes of his illnesses, and (2) find useful remedies.

On his "Road to Recovery," he found that there were many medical tests -- *which he lists in this book* **--- to detect and discover the underlying causes of his illnesses.**

If those **tests** had been performed at the beginning of his illnesses, Marc would have been spared many decades of pain, suffering, exhaustion and emotional problems.

On his "Road to Recovery," Marc found many **remedies, both traditional and non-traditional**, which helped him recover from his illnesses.

In this book, Marc shares what worked for him and others so that those who suffer from his illnesses may **suffer less and recover faster**.

Much of what Marc reveals is unusual or even controversial. But, he believes that the final chapter on the causes of these illnesses and their remedies have not yet been fully written.

Medical science has not yet provided definitive answers to the questions:

1. What causes CFS and Fibromyalgia?
2. Which remedies work best to alleviate the symptoms of those illnesses?

Marc believes that there is plenty of room for reasonable speculation about (1) what causes those illnesses, and (2) which treatments work best.

In response to those questions, **Marc shares what he knows has worked for him and what he believes will work for others.**

It is Marc's sincerest wish that his book will bring **relief** to those who suffer from these terrible illnesses as quickly as possible.

He truly desires that his book will provide **support, hope and good information** to patients, doctors, health care practitioners, and caregivers who help people who have these illnesses.

Lastly, it is Marc's greatest hope that his book will spur doctors, healers, health care practitioners, insurance companies and governmental agencies into giving **better care, testing and more money** to this group of most unfortunate patients.

1

My Story -
Big Challenges

I was born in 1948.   As of March, 2013, I will be 65 years old. Those who do not suffer from any of the illnesses which cause **"brain fog"** (cognitive impairment) will not be impressed by my ability to do this math.

But, those who have **cognition problems** (and there are millions of us who do) will appreciate that I am able to do the math so easily.   There was a long period of time when I couldn't do the math very easily. That ability was taken away from me by my illnesses. Truly, I have come a long way.

If you have "brain fog" from one or more of the illnesses about which I write, you will know what I am talking about. Otherwise, you will not.

If you have "brain fog," cognitive impairment or confusion, these neurological problems are sad, funny and overwhelming.

If you have these problems, you will understand how much I suffered when I was not able to do simple arithmetic, remember simple tasks or think straight. It was a profoundly, absurdly heart-wrenching few decades of my life.

You may notice that I have published this book using large print, margins and spaces between paragraphs. That was done intentionally.

I did these things because I am writing for a group of people, *which includes me*, who have *major difficulties reading, comprehending and remembering what we have just read.*

We must take extensive notes in the margins about what we have just read, or we won't be sure we just read it.

We need to write down our questions *immediately as they come to mind* or we will forget what we were just thinking about.

We need to underline and comment as we read so we can be sure we understood it.

We need to pause, think, ponder and write.

We need a lot of space in our books so we don't get confused.

I wrote this book using very simple language and easy to understand syntax. I wrote it that way because many of us have problem with cognition. We do not understand complex sentences. We need written communication to be simple and straight forward or we will not understand it.

I did not write this book for those who do not suffer from "brain fog" or cognitive impairment. I wrote it for those who do.

Those of you who have this condition will understand. Many have already expressed their appreciation for the way I have written this book.

Those who understand our plight and have empathy for us will understand why I wrote this book as I did as well.

But, those who don't have our condition or don't know people who have our condition, most likely won't understand our problems very well. It is just very difficult to imagine how it feels when you just can't think straight.

I learned a lot about our illnesses when I was co-chair of the Chronic Fatigue and Fibromyalgia Resource and Support Group of San Diego, California. I was co-chair for about 5 years in the late 1990's with Ms. Josephine Nost, who now lives near Tampa, Florida. She has been a great friend of mine for a very long time.

Our group met monthly. We invited a professional in the field of CFS or Fibromyalgia to speak to us. After the lecture, we socialized.

It was a loosely associated group of about 400 people, most of whom were chronically ill from CFS and Fibromyalgia. The others were caregivers for or supporters of persons with CFS or Fibromyalgia.

I learned that as a group, we have **unique problems**.

First, we are basically **invisible** to the general public.

To the average person, we look healthy and well, especially when we are out in public, which is usually only for a brief period of time. For the *average* person who is *disabled* with these illnesses, *we are only able to go out in public for an hour or two.*

However, there are truly tragic cases. Some of the worst cases in our group included men, women and young people who got up, showered and had to go right back to bed, *because washing exhausted them for the day.*

For those who can get up and get out for an hour or two, we look healthy, *except if you look into our eyes.* It is then that you would see the diminished signs of vitality which are masked by our wan smiles and cheerful countenance.

If you know what to look for, you would see that we are not well. But few people can see beyond our weak smiles and decently groomed appearances.

Few people know how to look into our eyes, beyond our tired smiles and weak voices.

As a result, our group *fooled most people* into believing they were feeling better than they actually were.

Unless you had one of these illnesses, then you knew. We all knew. *Because each of us was always sick, each of us was always tired.*

Second, I learned from our group members that people who do not have our illnesses *do not understand* our suffering and despair.

Each of us had tried to explain to our family, friends, doctors and healers about the horrible nature of our chronic exhaustion, continuous pain and genuine despair.

Each of us had tried to explain to our co-workers and bosses about our continuous pain and suffering. But, it was clear to me --- from my own experiences and from listening to others --- that *unless you had our illnesses, you just didn't "get it."*

When I was co-chair of the CFS and Fibromyalgia support group in San Diego, almost everyone started their conversation with what it was like to live with their illness.

Each person started with ---

how bad they felt; *how* much pain they were in; *how* tired they were; *how* little they could do; *how* bad their cognition was; *how* much physical, emotional and financial trouble they were in; *how* little understanding and support they received at home from their spouse, family and friends.

There were exceptions of course, but the general rule was that *we were alone* in our despair, suffering and grief.

Each of us carried on as best we could, but in general, very few of us received a sufficient amount of support from our friends and family.

Hardly anyone received sufficient financial support from the government, insurance company, generous friends or family members.

Too often, I heard how many of our members had been *abandoned* by their families, spouse, friends and bosses, because they could not give them the support they needed during their continuous times of pain, exhaustion, grief and despair.

Even after telling them that they didn't have to tell me their stories *because:*

> *I was one of them, and*
> *I knew what they were going through, and*
> *I had the same health challenges they had --*

they were so accustomed to being *misunderstood* by friends and family --- they felt *compelled* to tell me their stories and their complaints --- before moving on to *their real interests*, which **always** were ---

1. **What did my doctors find wrong with me?**

2. **What was I doing to get better?**

3. **Which doctors or healers could I recommend?**

4. **How could they get more money from the government or insurance company --- so they could pay their bills or go to more doctors?**

Then, our conversation really started. They asked me their most pressing questions:

What had I learned about how to get better and recover?

As a result of:

Their continuous pain and exhaustion caused by their illnesses,

Their overwhelming frustration caused by not knowing the causes of their illnesses,

Their hopelessness caused by not being able to remedy their chronic health problems,

Their depression caused by knowing they would never again be fully employed,

Their despair caused by constantly living in poverty and destitution,

Their continuing grief caused by having been abandoned by friends, family, government and insurance company,

The members of our group had *suicidal thoughts too often,* and sometimes *committed suicide.*

Sadly, too many good, decent and loving members of our group took their lives because life had become *unbearable* for them for too long.

It is for those who have been left without answers to their most basic questions about *(1) the causes of their illnesses,* and *(2) the remedies which could work best for them*; and,

It is for those who have been *left without hope* of *(1) discovering the causes of their illnesses,* or *(2) finding anything that might bring them some relief,* I have written this book.

To those who have our illnesses, let me say this:

For decades, I was where you are.

But for the Grace of God, and for some unknown reason, my life was spared, and I recovered.

After decades of suffering, by luck, I stumbled upon a few doctors, dentists and healers who had *new ideas* about what was causing my illnesses.

They had *new ideas* about how to fix me.

And, they were willing to risk the medical and dental establishments' wrath by using some *new or unorthodox techniques* to heal me.

And, as a result, I recovered.

I hope and pray that this book may bring you much needed relief as soon as possible on your "Road to Recovery."

Believe me,
my heart
is with you
forever.

2

Past Events,
Future Problems

I realize that many of my various health problems arose from events which happened a long time ago. I can remember events that caused significant health problems much later in life.

From having interviewed hundreds of patients with CFS and Fibromyalgia, I have seen that there are many similarities in our stories. I will use examples from my own life as a way of illustrating general principles which I believe to be true for most of us who suffer from these illnesses.

Head and Neck Injuries

Many persons with CFS and Fibromyalgia told me they had experienced *whiplash* injuries to their neck and head in the past. They said that someone or something had *hit them* hard on the head or neck where they blacked out or almost blacked out. Some said they had experienced significant *falls* which had caused concussions, significant head injuries, head or neck traumas, or black outs in the past.

I remember playing American tackle football on the ice near Cleveland, Ohio, during the late fall and winter up until the age of 18. I played with 6 to 12 other big, strapping young men. I did not wear a helmet or other protective equipment. I banged my head on the frozen earth while being tackled and tackling others.

It was great fun. But, looking back, my parents, teachers, doctors and I were not very smart about the long-term health problems that can be caused by having traumatic brain injuries. Now we are more aware of the consequences of traumatic brain injuries.

In the 1950's and 1960's, it was common for us kids to have "minor" head injuries which were caused by banging our heads on the ground when we tackled some guy or when we were tackled by the other guys. In those days, no one thought about the health consequences of having a concussion or other type of brain injury.

Fast forward to 2013. It is now recognized that a *traumatic brain injury may cause significant health problems years after injury was sustained.*

But, I believe it is still *unusual* for physicians, medical practitioners and other healers to associate traumatic brain injuries with CFS and Fibromyalgia.

Celiac disease

Celiac disease is the inability of the body to properly digest wheat and other grains which contain the same gluten. It is an auto-immune system disorder that affects the colon and small intestine.

It is now thought that celiac disease affects about 1% of the American population. It is believed that most people do not know that they have the disease, since many times the symptoms are subtle.

I believe celiac disease was an important cause of my severe exhaustion (CFS) and my severe pain (Fibromyalgia).

Celiac disease can cause other problems as well. It can cause mild to severe *constipation*. When I was four years old, for the first time, I had severe abdominal pain. That was caused because I was severely constipated.

To alleviate my abdominal pain, my caregivers gave me an enema. It worked fine. But, it should have been a BIG TIP OFF that I could not digest wheat. But it wasn't. *That important piece of my health puzzle was missed for more than five decades.* That was very bad for me. And it is very bad for people who are not properly diagnosed with celiac disease.

As a result of having celiac disease, I had abdominal pain. The pain was caused by having eaten white bread, which my body was not able to digest properly.

Because of celiac disease, the white bread became **wadded** up and **obstructed** my colon. That wad caused me to suffer *severe* abdominal pain.

Around the age of 36, I suffered from severe abdominal pain again. I had to be admitted to the

Emergency Room in a Washington, D.C. hospital because I was suffering so much pain.

X-rays revealed that I had a large wad of undigested food lodged in my intestines. I believe the undigested mass was composed of undigested wheat and other grains that had the same type of gluten I could not digest. Again, celiac disease proved to be very painful for me.

Celiac disease can also be subtle. It can tear you down. It can make you feel constantly weak, tired, exhausted and emotionally dysfunctional.

Celiac disease, I believe, can also wear out the villi in the intestines. Worn down villi can prevent the body from absorbing sufficient nutrients, which can make you feel weak, tired and exhausted.

In the extreme, celiac disease can also stunt a person's growth, as it did me.

When I was 12, I stopped growing taller after having been the second tallest boy in my class for years.

Even after extensive testing, my doctors did not discover the cause. They thought I had stopped growing because I had a dysfunctional pituitary gland. But, I believe I had stopped growing taller because I had celiac disease.

If I had known in 1960 that I had celiac disease, I would have avoided eating wheat and other foods that contained the same bad gluten.

By not eating wheat and those other grains containing the same harmful gluten, I would not have suffered most of the very severe health problems which occurred to me during my life.

In short, if I had been told at the age of twelve I had celiac disease, and I had been advised not to eat wheat and other foods which contained that bad gluten, I would not have suffered a lifetime of severe pain, chronic exhaustion, or accumulated most of those heavy metals which caused most of my big health problems.

But, that diagnosis was missed for five decades, and celiac disease ended up causing me to have many big health problems in my life.

Chronic Yeast and Fungal Infections

When I was twelve years old, I craved breads, cakes, ice cream, candy and cookies. Also, I was continuously fatigued and hypersensitive to cold. Finally, I became fatter, rounder and bloated.

Each of those symptoms should have indicated that I was suffering from chronic yeast and fungal infections. *But, together, they constituted a pattern that clearly indicated I was suffering from chronic yeast and fungal infections.*

Cognitive Impairment

When I was twelve years old, I had my first episode of "brain fog." Some call it "Fibro fog," too.

"Brain fog" is the condition where you just can't think straight. It is a form of cognitive impairment.

You have "brain fog" when you go to the refrigerator, open it, and cannot remember why you are there.

You have "brain fog" when you put your keys down, turn around, and can't remember where you put them.

You have "brain fog" when you drive through a stop sign that you've stopped at a thousand times before because you didn't realize it was there.

You have "brain fog" when you have read the same paragraph ten times in a row and still can't remember what you have just read.

You have "brain fog" when you have read the same sentence ten times in a row and can't understand what you have just read.

Everyone does one of these things once in a while. But, people with "brain fog" do these things almost every day, and sometimes many times a day.

Brain Fog Has Many Causes

"Brain fog" may be caused by a yeast or fungal infection which has spread throughout the body, including the brain.

It may be caused by a mycoplasma infection.

It may be caused by heavy metal toxicity, especially from mercury or lead.

It may be caused by a vitamin D3 deficiency.

It may be caused by a vitamin, mineral, amino acid, endocrine gland or enzyme deficiency.

It may be caused by all of the above, as it was in my case.

Emotional Problems

When I was fourteen, my emotions became hard to handle. I was tired and angry.

Obviously, adolescence played a large part, but, more was going on.

Yeast, fungus and mycoplasma can cause those kinds of emotional problems.

In addition, when I was fourteen, I became a very chatty person. That was a sign I had *mercury toxicity*.

In the 1800's, English workers pounded mercury by hand into felt hats to make them pliable.

Eventually, mercury toxicity made the workers unable to stop chatting. They were described as being "mad." Hence the expressions "Mad as a Hatter" or "Mad Hatter" came about.

Emotional Outbursts

When I was fifteen, my emotional levels were very high. I was highly charged with anger. Emotional problems can be caused by accumulation of heavy metals in the liver, mycoplasma infection, yeast or fungus infections, alcoholism or hypoglycemia.

Short-term Memory Dysfunction

When I was fifteen, my short-term memory became seriously problematic. It became much worse by the time I was sixteen.

At 15, I tried to memorize lines for a short school play. I rehearsed and practiced by repeating them many, many times. But, even after 100's of repetitions, I could not remember my lines.

By the time I was 16, I couldn't recall what I had been trying to memorize just a few minutes before. No matter how much I practiced, I could not make anything stick in my memory. French class was my "Waterloo" (pun intended).

Depression

By the time I was 18, I had my first episode of a major depression. Thankfully, the depression was fairly mild. However, for the next few years, until I was 25, it was manageable but constantly influencing my life.

Weight Gain

From the ages of 26 until 38, (1974 until 1986), I gained 116 pounds. I went from 130 to 246 lbs. (I was 5'8"). I went from being skinny to morbidly obese.

No one understood what caused me to eat so much food. *I used to be hungrier after I ate a meal than before I started.*

I believe that **when I started to eat, the yeast and fungus came alive and demanded I feed them more food**. They are beasts. They caused me to gain a lot of weight.

Chronic Exhaustion

At twenty-six, in 1974, I was "burned out". My doctor ordered me to rest more and work less. He ordered that I work only part time. He thought I was overworked, but that was not true.

I worked as a business and real estate attorney. My job consisted of preparing routine paper work. My job was not stressful or tiring.

I worked 7 hours per day and only five days per week. That was not much for a young attorney. My doctor and I did not know it then, but I was suffering from a full blown case of CFS.

CFS

From the time I was 26 through 43 years old, (1974 through 1991) I was totally exhausted. From the time I was 41 through 43, I was sleeping 20 hours per day. Watching TV, reading a book, or grocery shopping made me exhausted and fall asleep. Everything put me to sleep.

Fibromyalgia

When I was 39 years old, (1987), I developed severe, chronic pain all over my body, but especially in my legs. It was horribly painful, particularly at night.

I needed sedatives to make me stay asleep. Otherwise, the pain in my legs would awaken me every two hours, and I would not get any good sleep.

Despair

By 1991, at the age of 43, after 17 years of being chronically exhausted, and after enduring 4 years of constant pain, I was in total despair.

I was in *total despair* because I had no hope of recovering. I believed there were no remedies or cures for my health problems. I was *without any hope* of remission. I was in total despair.

I believed I was only going to get worse. I had come to the point of having endured enough pain in my life, and I was ready put an end to my suffering. I set a date --- six months and two days in the future --- which was the exact day my wife would be legally assured of receiving all the life insurance benefits I had purchased for her two years before. After two years, the life insurance company had to pay all benefits to her and could not contest the policy even if I committed suicide.

Despite being married to the most wonderful, charming, beautiful woman on the planet, my despair had reached its limit. My pain and exhaustion had become too great to bear.

Despite living in a wonderful new home in a very lovely city, having good relationships with friends and family, I was without hope.

I was constantly exhausted, chronically in pain, always hungry and angry, confused, bitter, sad, depressed, brain fogged, cognitively and short-term memory impaired. I was totally worn out.

By 1991, I was no longer able to work as a lawyer, even part time, because I was too tired and too brain fogged to think straight.   I could not remember facts.   My short-term memory had been destroyed.

By 1991, I was so tired that I could barely watch TV, read a book, listen to music or go to the supermarket before I fell asleep.   By 1991, I was sleeping 20 hours per day.

By 1991, I often suffered from some weird, strange malady.   Suddenly, without warning or cause, my hands would swell, double their size, and itch like crazy.

Suddenly and without cause, my stomach blew up to twice its normal size.

Suddenly and without cause, a dozen hives popped out on my stomach and abdomen.

At night, my legs had so much pain I had to take a sedative (Klonopin) to keep myself asleep for at least 6 hours. Otherwise, I would be awakened by the pain throughout the night and never get a full night's rest

Every morning, I woke up more tired than when I went to bed. I was miserable.

My only hope of escaping from my chronic pain and exhaustion was to commit suicide. Only the Will of God kept me from completing that last, final, desperate, selfish act of obtaining eternal relief.

But, in late1991, my luck began to change. Dr. Gary Shima, MD diagnosed me as suffering from the toxic effects of having *heavy metal toxicity* and *immune system dysfunction*.

Those diagnoses explained in large part why I was totally exhausted, in such great pain, and so emotionally distraught for so many years.

Later, I was diagnosed with *celiac disease.*

That diagnosis explained why:

    1.   **I** had *stopped growing* when I was twelve years old,

    2.   **I** was so constipated throughout my lifetime,

3.   I could *not properly digest and absorb* the nutrients from my food,

4.   I could *not eliminate toxic heavy metals* from my body.

During the next two decades, *other important diagnoses* arose, which explained why I was so tired, in so much pain, and so emotionally distraught.

During the next twenty years, I was diagnosed with having:

1.   **hypothyroidism,** which caused my constant fatigue and poor metabolic functioning,

2.   **neuropathy,** which caused my Fibromyalgia (pain),

3.   **hypersensitivity to light, sound, and odors,** which caused my exhaustion and pain,

4. **kidney disorder,** which caused my Fibromyalgia (pain),

5. **yeast and fungus infections,** which caused my exhaustion, huge stomach bloating, obesity, *hypoglycemia*, "brain fog" and balance problems,

6. **virus and bacterial infections,**

7. **flukes (worms),**

8. **psoriasis,**

9. **depression,**

10. **mycoplasma fermentans incognitus infection.**

Mycoplasma fermentans incognitus is a Biological Weapon of Mass Destruction (WMD).

A patent has been issued to a scientist who worked for the U.S. government at Fort Dietrich, Maryland.

It was created with the intention of making anyone who becomes infected by that WMD totally anemic and emotionally unstable.

Dr. Garth Nicolson, Ph.D. testified before Congress on his findings about this mycoplasma.

He believes that the above mycoplasma contaminated the U.S. soldiers during the first Gulf War, and is the **primary cause** of the **Gulf War Syndrome**.

I have written how I twice cured myself of mycoplasma in a later section of this book.

The general form of mycoplasma is a terrible pathogen. It *robs the body of energy* and causes chronic exhaustion.

It makes the body weak by invading the red blood cells, and then destroys the cells' ability to use oxygen, iron and vitamin B-12.

Without oxygen, iron and vitamin B-12, I became chronically weak, tired, exhausted, anemic and in great pain.

When mycoplasma *dies-off*, it creates major *emotional problems*. The die-off can cause severe bouts of anger, rage and hostility. In addition, the die off can cause severe pain (Fibromyalgia).

On my "Road to Recovery," I was diagnosed with other illnesses as well. They were:

1. **sleep apnea**
2. **vitamin D3 deficiency**
3. **enzyme deficiency**

4. **adrenal exhaustion**
5. **essential fatty acid deficiency**
6. **DHEA deficiency**

Each of the above illnesses caused chronic exhaustion and brain fog.

It was a very long and exhausting process to discover the causes of my illnesses, and then to use various remedies to recover from them.

It took decades to discover the pieces of my medical puzzle, and then put the pieces into a coherent order.

The inter-relationship of these illnesses was *not* explained in any textbooks.

Much of what was discovered had to be improvised by my doctors as I progressed along my "Road to Recovery."

Good testing and common sense played a large part in discovering what was wrong with me.

Once the causes of my illnesses were discovered, the remedies were not too hard to figure out.

This book is a compilation of what I learned from my doctors, health care practitioners, healers, and other patients who had similar illnesses.

It is also a compilation of my opinions, which are based upon my own experiences and the experiences of others.

During the 38 years it took me to regain my health, I developed various theories about the causes and remedies of my illnesses.

I hope that by sharing my information, experiences, ideas and thoughts with those who suffer from these illnesses, they will find relief quicker, easier and cheaper.

I hope they will receive better care from their doctors, health care providers, healers, caregivers, support system, insurance company and government.

**To those who suffer
From these illnesses:
I wish you the *best* of luck:
That you quickly *discover*
The *causes* of your illnesses,
And you *find*
The very best *remedies*,
Right now.**

3

Helping Others
Improved My Health

In the course of learning about my illnesses, I shared my knowledge with other patients and the 100 or so doctors, healers and health care practitioners who were helping me.

I found that
the more I shared,
at my own expense,
the more I recovered.

I discovered that
the *more I gave* to others,
with a genuine wish
to help those who were less fortunate,
the *more* my health improved.

That was the *most* important lesson
I learned when I was so ill.

In addition, I came to believe that the following sayings are True.

What goes 'round, comes 'round.

As you do unto others,
it will be done unto you.

The law of karma is beyond doubt.

Over the years, I have shared these lessons with many people.

So I take this opportunity to share them with you.

First and foremost,
I consider them to be that important.

4

Acceptance and Trust
In the Higher Power

When I was very sick, I had the time and inclination to call upon God as my Higher Power for help.

I was helpless when confronted by my overwhelming illnesses.

I was left with only my faith in God and that my life was proceeding just as it should be, despite not going as I had previously planned.

I went from being the typical young American lawyer, who was full of himself and his self-assured future success, to completely surrendering to my fate that I was living with a situation where I was completely helpless.

I had no other choice in the matter because I literally could not do anything else. I couldn't read, watch TV, work or play without falling asleep.

By 1991, my life had been reduced to eating, sleeping and breathing. I could no longer work, play or do productive things. I was that sick.

I lived day-by-day, prayerfully, waiting and hoping that someday I might get well.

But, in my time of total sickness, I was still able to help others --- by listening to them, making suggestions, giving support, making them laugh, and taking care of my family's daily needs.

I came to realize that my future was no longer under my control because I was barely able to survive.

Over time, I accepted my fate and the fact that I had no control over my future.

I had to turn control of my life over to God. I could only wait for a miracle, or I was going to die.

I learned not to think about how I was going to make a living or control my destiny.

During those decades of great illness, I learned to surrender to the Grace of God, and believe that He had a reason for my becoming totally disabled.

I found it was good for my state of mind if I added a good amount of faith to my daily routine. That helped me get through the day.

It was comforting to me to believe that God had some kind of plan for my life, even though His plan was not obvious to me.

Over time, I found myself becoming more compassionate toward those who were ill or less fortunate.

I could relate to them because I was now one with them. I could resonate with their lives and their stories because I too was one of the less fortunate.

I could see that my illnesses were making me a more compassionate person, even as they kept me from earning a lot of money, power, fame and prestige.

I took comfort in my personal growth. I had no other choice.

It was nice to know that science had shown that prayer worked to heal people quicker.

But, it felt better to know that I was getting closer to God as I lay sick on my bed, day after day, night after night.

Surrender to my fate brought me peace of mind, especially as I endured great pain, exhaustion and suffering.

I found that it was best if I stopped worrying about the future, and put my faith in God.

I found wonderment, and even some joy, in my life's journey -- even if was not the kind of life I had planned when I was a young attorney with great ambitions.

After a few years, I accepted my new reality. I surrendered to the idea that I was no longer going to be an attorney who was going to have great fame and fortune.

Instead, I saw myself as a person who was destined to become more compassionate and who had a lot of unusual but useful health information to share with doctors, healers and those in need.

I became fascinated by my transformation from attorney to healer. I found happiness when I accepted my fate, my destiny and my karma.

Being ill, I realized, was my life's adventure. Every day, I was on a very dangerous adventure, trying to find what ailed me, and then, to find a cure.

It was a fascinating journey because every day brought a surprise of finding that my doctors had discovered that I suffered from a new illness.

My life became my own personal drama, which was also fascinating.

At all times, I knew that the end of my adventure might result in my death. I was that sick.

Or, the adventure might somehow lead me to recovery.

I had no idea how my drama was going to end. All I knew was that with God, all things were possible. And only He could save me.

I began to take each day as it came, one day at a

time, one step at a time. I had no hope, but I had gone beyond total despair.

Without hope, daily, I waited for God to work His miracles on me. I prayed. And, I went on, day by day.

My life became my own personal drama. I became the main character in my own story of life and death. Interestingly, I did not know how the story would end.

In the context of my life being a life and death struggle for survival, my story became very interesting to me.

Each day a new piece of information was added to my health puzzle. Patterns were starting to be revealed.

Almost daily, my doctors revealed new discoveries about my illnesses. That process gave me hope and interest. I had passed beyond the time of my great despair.

I came to understand that God was the playwright of my drama.

I came to know that my life was completely and totally in His hands.

I came to know that I would live or die based only on what He ordained for me.

I watched myself go through my illnesses as an audience watched a play. Except, I was the main character in my own drama. And, I was the audience as well.

Since I had no idea of how my drama would end,

it was very interesting to me. It was really very dramatic to me.

I came know that no matter how much I wanted to know the conclusion of my life's drama, it was not going to be revealed until God decided it was time for me to know that information.

I came to understand these Truths:

1. **Life is on a "Need to Know" basis.**

2. **When God Wanted Me to Know Something, He Will Reveal It.**

3. **Life is on His Schedule.**

4. **The Truth Will Not Be Revealed Before Its Time.**

I stopped demanding God reveal the end of my drama to me. I stopped asking when or if I would recover. Instead, I relaxed.

I tried to remember that my health issues were just another episode in my life's drama.

I tried to find enjoyment in each day's events, no matter how painful or exhausting.

I realized that to stay happy, I had to stop worrying about the future.

I realized that worrying about my health would not change the present, past or future.

I realized that I should not worry about the future because it would not make me feel better. It would only make me feel worse.

So, I tried to limit worrying about how my drama would end.

I realized that I should give up getting upset about not being able to pursue my prior goals. That was the past. That was not what God wanted me to do.

I tried to relax and took one day at a time.

I surrendered to my fate.

I surrendered to the fact that my life I was literally in God's hands.

I surrendered control of my life to Him. He was the absolute captain of my ship.

That meant if He wanted me to get better, He had to do it. My life was under his control.

That meant if He didn't want me to get better, I wouldn't.

It was up to Him to heal me. If I were to get better, it would be on His terms, on His schedule and in His way.

Over time, I surrendered to my fate of being totally disabled, and I made peace with the Lord.

As I forced myself to change my point of view from being an ego-centric, Western, materialistic man to a spiritually-centered, surrendered-unto-God yogi man, a few very interesting things began to happen.

Insights came to me which seemed profoundly important.

One insight was that I had to go through these illnesses in order to gain these insights.

Another insight was that it was my calling to be sick so that I could learn and understand some very basic spiritual truths.

Over time, deeper spiritual truths became apparent to me.

I began to understand that to reach my highest happiness, it was necessary to make my heart fill with love and compassion at all times.

I began to understand that I was here to serve God and to serve others in love, peace and harmony.

I began to understand that
each of us is here on Planet Earth to learn

To love God, and
To love each other.

I began to learn that

Love is Caring and Sharing.

Falling in love is bio-karmic-
electro-magnetic attraction.

I laughed. I realized that prior to my illnesses, I had heard those words, but had not understood their meaning.

As I lay chronically exhausted and in severe pain, day after day, year after year, those words became living testaments which resonated in my heart and soul.

I laughed at what pain and suffering it took to make me realize their more significant meaning.

I began to understand that we humans grow wiser through suffering.

That was a truth which became very apparent to me over time.

I laughed at how simple these Truths were.

I began to understand that we humans grow more mature by "Taking up Our Individual Crosses," and by sacrificing pleasure for the sake of spiritual gain.

I began to learn that irony and paradox were the touchstones of Truth.

I began to learn that the books of Job and Genesis were very important to me.

I began to realize that those insights would not have come if I had I been healthy and worked as a business attorney.

I began to realize that my illnesses had given me the time and opportunity to commune with God.

I began to realize that He had given me the time and opportunity to commune with Him.

I began to realize that my illnesses had given me the chance to enter into the Spirit of God.

I began to realize that my illnesses had given me the time and opportunity to discover what I needed to know about the meaning of life.

**We are All
Angels in Training.**

and

**Planet Earth Is
Boot Camp for the Soul.**

I began to realize that those insights had given me great peace of mind, humor, fun, joy, love, compassion and a desire to be of greater service to others, despite my body being very sick and I was not very successful financially.

I began to realize that during my illnesses, God had the time to work His magic on me --- and was *transforming me into a wiser, more compassionate humane human being.*

I considered that a fair trade. I took on a sick body in exchange for an improved heart and soul.

I began to think that my illnesses were a blessing.

I began to realize that my illnesses had:

Refined my soul,

Allowed me to purify my thoughts,

Permitted me to enter into the Kingdom of Heaven in order to receive greater understanding,

Made me into a much better, happier person.

I began to realize that having these kinds of insights made me very happy.

I began to be happy that my life turned out the way it did, illnesses and all.

I began to realize that I still struggled with my desire for more money.

I began to realize that taming the inner demons is part of the process of becoming more humane.

For all of the above, I have become grateful and happy, despite having experienced the physical, mental and emotional crucibles of suffering for a long period of time.

I began to see that my illnesses had helped me grow wiser, more loving, and more compassionate, because I had experienced so much suffering over such a long period of time.

I began to see that when I was young, becoming a more humane person was not something I thought was of much value.

I began to see that becoming a more *humane person* was the only thing of value, and becoming a more *humane person* was the only thing worth striving for.

I began to see how we humans are deluded into pursuing false goals.

It's funny that I didn't see all these things until I had been ill for a very long time.

I began to think that all of the above was amazing.

My heart began to be constantly filled with joy, because God had replaced the old selfish me with a more loving and compassionate me.

I found myself thinking:

*When I am Centered in the
Universe of Love, and
You are Centered in the
Universe of Love,
Then, We Are Truly Blessed and One.*

Namaste

5

Chronic Fatigue Syndrome (CFS)
Has No Medically Defined Cause or Causes

Chronic Fatigue Syndrome (CFS) is just what it says it is. It is a syndrome. Therefore, there are no specific underlying causes for the illness.

However, I found from my own experience and from speaking with others that there are many similar causes of the Chronic Fatigue Syndrome. I discuss them in this book.

The Chronic Fatigue Syndrome is a *descriptive* diagnosis. It is a diagnosis that is reached by the doctor only after he or she has *excluded from possibility through testing and diagnosis* every other illness that looks like CFS.

There are certain characteristics of CFS, but they are not causes. If the patient's illness has those characteristics, but his or her doctor cannot find any specific cause for the chronic exhaustion and other symptoms, then the doctor gives the patient a diagnosis of "Chronic Fatigue Syndrome."

For example, after testing reveals that the patient does *not* suffer from things like lupus, cancer, herpes, mycoplasma, hypothyroidism heart disease, HIV, Epstein-Barr, sleep apnea, mercury toxicity or depression, the doctor will diagnose the patient as suffering from CFS.

If the patient is told by the doctor that he or she has CFS, it means that the patient suffers from chronic exhaustion plus a few other symptoms, but the doctor does not know the cause. That is the reason CFS is called a "syndrome."

Being *diagnosed* with CFS tells the patient only what he or she *doesn't* have. That may be comforting, but it does *not* tell the patient what he or she *does* have.

There is **big problem** with being diagnosed with CFS ---

If the patient doesn't know what is causing his or her chronic exhaustion, it is very difficult --- or almost impossible --- to find a cure or an appropriate remedy.

6

Chronic Fatigue Syndrome
Is Not Depression

CFS looks like chronic depression, but it is not. There are major *differences* that distinguish the two disorders.

There are many *similarities* between CFS and chronic depression. Both types of patients are without much energy, stay at home very often, and don't seem to be able to do much.

Someone can have CFS and depression at the same time. They are *not mutually exclusive* illnesses.

However, there are some very important *differences* between a person with CFS and one who has chronic depression.

First, CFS patients generally *do not react favorably to anti-depressant medications* unless they suffer from depression as well.

Often, patients with CFS report very bad side effects from taking anti-depressant medications. This does not generally occur with people suffering from depression.

Bad side effects occur with CFS patients because *CFS is not a serotonin problem.*

Second, CFS patients, most often, *cannot tolerate exercise* without becoming seriously ill. The bad side effects from exercise may last a day, many days or even a couple of weeks.

On the other hand, patients suffering from *chronic depression* generally report that exercise *helps* them feel much better.

Quite often, a patient who suffers from depression will swear that his or her exercise program is medically necessary to maintain his or her physical and mental health. Patients who suffer from CFS do not find that exercise improves their mental health or moods at all.

CFS patients do **not** get a *"runner's high."* We wonder,

> **"Why do other people enjoy exercise**
> **so much?"**

because it is *not* an enjoyable part of our life's experience (if it ever was).

When CFS patients exercise too much, we often become very ill. That is radically different from patients who suffer from chronic depression.

Third, CFS and Fibromyalgia patients *actively seek out advice* from many doctors and healers when we are searching for causes, cures and remedies.

We actively search the internet for the latest developments about our illnesses.

We read magazines and newspaper articles about our illnesses. We join groups to discuss our illnesses with others who have our problems.

We are very proactive when trying to recover until we become overwhelmed physically, emotionally or financially.

Then, we become reclusive because we no longer have enough energy or other resources to keep going.

Patients with CFS and Fibromyalgia *actively search* for many different kinds of doctors and health care professionals from a variety of sources, while patients with chronic depression do this much less.

Patients with CFS and Fibromyalgia *go to many* health food stores, health conventions and alternative healers, while patients with chronic depression do this much less.

Patients with CFS and Fibromyalgia use the opinions of *many* doctors, healers, and health care practitioners and will try many different kinds of remedies, while patients with chronic depression will seek out the opinion of just one or two doctors, take just one or two pills, and if that does not work, will do nothing more.

Patients who suffer from CFS and Fibromyalgia tend to be *proactive* in their recovery process, while those who suffer from chronic depression do much less. I exaggerate to make these points.

Fourth, chronic depression may be caused by excessive amounts of *cortisol*. Medications may help reduce excessive amounts of cortisol and relieve that kind of depression.

CFS is *not caused by excessive amounts of cortisol*, so those kinds of medications do not eliminate CFS, unless CFS is also caused by yeast and fungus infections. Then, there may be an overlap between those illnesses. Some medications may alleviate both sets of problems.

Many doctors are not aware of some of these differences. It is an area of medicine where doctors may need to use more caution to avoid causing additional harm to CFS and Fibromyalgia patients.

7

Chronic Fatigue Syndrome
is Heavy Metal Toxicity

After 17 years of disabling exhaustion, I was diagnosed with suffering from the toxic effects of heavy metal accumulation. I suffered from excessive amounts of mercury, lead, nickel, vanadium and cadmium which were stored in my body.

Each of these heavy metals is very toxic, very poisonous, and all of them had accumulated far in excess of the maximum safe level.

After 17 years of becoming progressively worse, my doctor and his assistants discovered that I was being poisoned to death on a daily basis by these heavy metals.

The basic effects from heavy metal poisoning were as follows:

disabling exhaustion

continuous confusion

brain fog

severe pain

emotional disorders

hypersensitivities to sound, light and odors

unrestful sleep

post exercise dysfunction

malabsorption

digestion and elimination dysfunction

immune system dysfunction

yeast and fungal infections

viral and bacterial infections

mycoplasma infection

endocrine system dysfunction

My doctor performed **three preliminary medical tests** to determine if I had heavy metal toxicity.

First, I had a hair test;

Second, I had a live blood cell analysis;

Third, I had an electronic wave machine test called the "Interro," which analyzed by computer my body's responses to the various electrical impulses which were sent through the electrodes I held in my hands.

Each of these **preliminary tests** accurately identified that I had high levels of heavy metals in my body.

After all of that preliminary testing, finally, my doctor performed a **standard medical test** using a **chelating** agent to determine the precise level of heavy metals in my body.

That standardized test conclusively proved I was suffering from the toxic effects of excessive amounts of lead, nickel, mercury, vanadium and cadmium, all heavy metals, which had accumulated to excessively large amounts in my body.

Questions:

(1)   **Where did I get those heavy metals?**
(2)   **Why did I store them?**

Answers:

(1)   I **absorbed** the heavy metals from the **environment**.

(2)   Since my colon was **clogged up** from the effects of **celiac disease**, I **stored them**.

(3)   I **stored** them **because it was too dangerous for my body to discharge them** from my liver into my colon, **because they would end up in my bloodstream, thus poisoning my body and brain.**

I absorbed *heavy metals* from the environment.

When I was growing up, from 1948 to 1969, there were no significant environmental regulations. It was a time in the U.S. before there was the federal Clean Air Act and the Clean Water Act.

I absorbed *mercury* from the environment.

I absorbed mercury from the fillings that were used to fill the cavities in my teeth. I absorbed mercury when I polished dimes with it when I was a child. I absorbed mercury when I used mercurochrome to disinfect cuts I received when I was a child.

I absorbed mercury by breathing mercury contaminated fumes which were emitted from the coal burning electric power plants in my city.

I absorbed *lead* from the environment.

Lead was in the paint that was on the wooden slats that kept me safe in my crib as an infant. I teethed on those wooden slats, ate the paint, and absorbed the lead.

Lead was in the paint that coated the No. 2 orange pencils that I used in elementary school. I chewed on those pencils, ate the paint, and absorbed the lead.

Lead was in the tap water. It leached into the water from the solder that that was used to weld the copper water pipes together.

Lead was in gasoline, both of which I breathed and absorbed.

I loved breathing those gasoline fumes. I *loved* inhaling those fumes because my body was substituting the oil in the gasoline fumes for essential fatty acids which were deficient in my diet and body.

My body was making that substitution in order to stay alive and grow. It was a short-term fix, but it caused long-term problems.

I absorbed *nickel* from the environment.

Nickel was in my stainless steel cookware, my stainless steel cutlery, and in my stainless steel braces, which were on my teeth for six years.

Nickel was in my French horn's stainless steel mouthpiece, which I played almost every day for six years.

I absorbed *vanadium* and *cadmium* from the environment.

Vanadium was in our air. I breathed it and absorbed it. It came from the steel mills which were upwind. It came from our electric power plant which was upwind.

I absorbed cadmium from cigarette smoke. It was absorbed first-hand when I smoked a little, and I absorbed it second-hand when my parents smoked in my presence.

I breathed and ate those heavy metals, and my body did not excrete them well enough to keep me healthy.

Instead, my cells and organs absorbed them. As a result, over time I became very sick from absorbing too many heavy metals. Unfortunately, I was an **absorber**.

Everyone breathes and eats some heavy metals from the environment, but their bodies do not absorb them very much. Instead, their bodies excrete them. They are **excreters**. Therefore, most people do not suffer the problems I did.

Because I had **celiac disease**, my body did not excrete those heavy metals. *Instead, my body* **stored** *and* **absorbed** them. The result was I became very sick with CFS, Fibromyalgia and depression.

After 17 years of being highly dysfunctional, and without any diagnosis, and without any hope of recovery, I became suicidal. Without hope, I saw no point in living. Suicide was settled in my mind.

I literally challenged God, "If You don't want me to come home, You had better fix me."

Surprisingly, He did.

Obviously, He had other plans for me, and He wasn't about to let me commit suicide.

Let me finish this section by sharing one of my favorite ironic, humorous bits of truth.

"If you want to make God laugh,
tell Him *your* plans!"

I told Him my plans in December, 1990, when I said I was going to commit suicide --- and He laughed.

Over the next 22 years, He caused me to recover my health, very slowly and with great effort. But, recover I did.

Looking back, my plans that day didn't work out. In fact, *none of the plans in my life* worked out.

But, I see now that I'm much happier because none of them worked out!

Go figure!

I have learned that:

Irony and Paradox Rule.

8

Chelation and Colonics
Saved My Life

After my doctor determined I was suffering from the toxic effects of having accumulated excessive amounts of heavy metals in my body, the obvious course of action was to remove the heavy metals.

He recommended that I start on a program of using chelating agents to remove the heavy metals. In late 1991, at the age of 43, I began to use chelation.

Chelation is a medical procedure where a chemical agent is put into a body through a vein in the arm by a slow, intravenous drip over a 3 or 4 hour period.

The chemical then binds with the heavy metals as well as all other electrically charged particles in the body.

The body then excretes the heavy metals and all other electrically charged particles, called **electrolytes**, during urination.

There is a potential problem with chelation. When the electrolytes are removed, the electrical system of the body, including the brain and nerves, are put at risk from depletion. Over time, the body may suffer harm.

To avoid potential problems, electrolytes in the form of minerals are put back into the body by using an IV drip.

In fact, I had three IV's per week. Two were chelations and one was an electrolyte replacement.

After the first six weeks, I had 12 chelations and 6 electrolyte replacements. I felt great. I thought my doctor had found *the* cure. However, that was not to be true.

After the ninth week, I had 18 chelations and 9 electrolyte replacements, but my body had become too weak and exhausted to continue.

My doctor was mystified. He did not understand what was going wrong. So, we decided to stop the chelation treatment.

He recommended that I use colon hydrotherapy (hereafter called a **"colonic"**) to flush out the heavy metals from my body.

In late January 1992, at the age of 43, I had my first colonic.

I was amazed because it worked so well.

From the first colonic, I felt great relief. I was amazed because my body did not suffer any bad side effects like I experienced with chelations. Most importantly, I felt great afterwards.

Because I had felt such great relief from the first colonic, I decided to continue.

After each colonic, I felt wonderful. Plus, there were no negative side effects. The proof was in the pudding. Colonics made me feel better.

During each colonic, I could **see and feel** toxins leave my body.

*I felt the toxic load in my body being reduced during and after each colonic. I knew that the level of poisons in my body was going down, and **I was going to recover.***

During and after each colonic, I felt I was witnessing a miracle. I watched my vitality and life slowly return to me in health, joy and happiness.

I was constantly filled with awe, happiness and gratitude during those amazing years which I gratefully shared with my wife.

During each colonic I literally *felt* the toxins leave my body. Whenever the toxins were released from my body, I felt the stress. I used to break into a sweat and became light-headed from the toxic release.

Also, I *saw* the water --- which passed out of my body and then through the tube on the colonic machine --- *change color*.

I saw the water turn *from clear to bright neon yellow* when the heavy metal toxins were released from my body. Sometimes I saw the water turn *from clear to bright pink* when lead was released from my body.

My recovery detox process was very slow.

During the years 1 and 2, I did three colonics per week.

For years 3 and 4, I did two colonics per week.

For years 5 and 6, I did one colonic per week.

For years 7 and 8, I did one colonic every two weeks.

It took almost 9 years for my body to release all of the toxins I had accumulated during my lifetime. It was a very long, slow, laborious process.

I learned to honor my body's time schedule of release and recovery. I could not do it faster or I would have hurt myself. I had to become a very patient patient (joke/pun) to regain my health.

Since the 9th year, I have one colonic every four or five weeks because I have a body which accumulates toxins.

Because I take many medicines for various unrelated health issues, they can cause an accumulation of toxins during the month. I continue to use colonics on a monthly basis to remove the accumulation of those toxins in order to continue feeling great.

9

The Colonic Process

In a nutshell, the process can be described as follows: The colonic infused my colon with water and stimulated my liver to dump its stored toxics into the water. The toxin filled water was deposited into my colon and was then removed from my colon through the use of the hydrotherapy "colonic" machine.

To help stimulate my liver, the colon hydro-therapist used her hand or a vibrating machine to pump moderately on my abdomen just above my liver while I was filled with water during the colonic.

That palpitation stimulated my liver to release the toxins into the water, which was then dumped into my colon. Then, my colon dumped the water out of my body through the colonic machine.

As the water left my body, I could see it passing through the tube which was on the colonic machine.

When my liver dumped the toxins, the water changed color. Most often, the water went from clear to neon yellow. Sometimes, it went from clear to neon red.

As the toxins left my body, I felt the effects of the release. It caused sweating for a few minutes and light-headedness. But, those symptoms passed quickly.

However, the benefits were so great that the minor side effects were soon forgotten. After the colonic, I felt amazingly good. Feeling great made me want to do it again.

Soon, the process became repetitive. Over the next couple of days, more toxins were released by the cells in my body, and those toxins were then stored in my liver.

The next colonic caused my liver to release those newly stored toxins into the water. That water was again dumped into my colon. Again, those toxins were passed out of my colon into the water, and the water was eliminated through the colonic machine.

After 9 years, my body released all the toxins which had accumulated during my lifetime.

As the amount of toxins in my body lessened, I slowly regained my health.

Colonics, indeed, saved my life.

10

Colonic Discoveries

During the process, my doctor, my colon hydro-therapist and I made some startling discoveries.

1.   When I used **ultrasound** on my liver or teeth during a colonic, it *greatly increased peristalsis*. I called that a **"sonic colonic."**

2.   When I used various colored **lights**, but especially **blue light,** which was emitted from a low powered cool laser, or **infrared light**, on the liver or teeth during a colonic, it *greatly increased peristalsis*. I called that a **"photonic colonic."**

Peristalsis is the muscular process by which the body moves food in the throat, through the stomach, the small and large intestines, and finally removes solid waste from the body.

3. *When I used ultrasound or light during a colonic, it greatly increased the amount of waste matter I released during my colonic.*

4. *When I used ultrasound or light during a colonic, it greatly increased the amount of toxins and heavy metals and lymph material I released during my colonic.*

5. *My body **dumped toxins from my lymph system** during a colonic.*

11

Signs of Lymph Drainage

First, lymph material was seen going through the clear glass tube on the colonic machine. It looked like bits and pieces of light, wispy mucus.

Second, when the lymph material was released from my body, I experienced severe sweating.

Third, when the lymph discharged its toxins, there was a fair amount of pain. The pain was worse than that which occurred when the liver released its toxins.

Fourth, when the lymph release stopped, all of the above symptoms stopped, and *I felt wonderful.*

Because of the great health benefits I received from colonics, I lovingly share my motto with you:

A Clean Colon
Is a Happy Colon!

12

Additional Benefits
from Colonics

1.   **Colonics promote beautiful skin.** When toxins are removed from the body, which may have accumulated from smoking cigarettes, the skin appears clear, radiant and youthful into old age.

Think of the film and stage actress Mae West and her beautiful skin. It is my understanding that she used colonics regularly.

The skin is the fourth largest organ of detoxification in the body, after the intestines, lungs and lymph system. When toxins have been removed from the body, the skin is relieved from processing their removal, and is under much less stress. The result is more beautiful looking skin.

2. **Colonics promote weight loss and size reduction.** When I removed excess waste matter from my body, I lost weight and reduced my size.

When toxins and poisons were removed from my body, my cells retained less fluid and shrank in size and volume. The result was I lost weight and reduced size.

My food metabolism and assimilation were improved through the use of colonics. I required less food to maintain my energy and vitality. The result was I lost weight and reduced size.

3. **Colonics can reduce low back pain.** When excess waste matter accumulates in the colon, the nerves in the lower back can be chronically stimulated. That can lead to low back pain. When excess waste matter is removed through colonics, lower back pain can be reduced.

4. **Colonics promote lymph system drainage and cleaning.** Colonics help stimulate the body to remove waste matter from the lymph system. Colonics also clear the colon so the body can safely discharge this highly toxic waste matter from the lymph system.

*The **lymph system** is the garbage dump of the body for toxic waste.* The lymph system surrounds each of the cells, and the cells dump their waste into the lymph system. The lymph system is very large. It has three times the volume of the blood supply. **When it became full of toxins, I became exhausted**.

A **lymph system** is difficult to clean. Colonics are one method of promoting the expulsion of toxic material from the lymph system.

There are other **ways to stimulate the lymph system** to help rid itself of toxins and waste matter.

Some methods are:

- Vigorous marching
- Pumping your arms and legs up and down
- Jumping up and down on a trampoline
- Jumping up and down without a trampoline
- Vigorous massaging the lymph nodes
- Using Light Therapy on Lymph Nodes

13

Chronic Fatigue Syndrome
Has Many Causes

1. CFS is Yeast or Fungus Overgrowth or Die-Off
2. CFS is Immune System Dysfunction
3. CFS is a Weak Immune System
4. CFS is Leaky Gut Syndrome
5. C FS is Allergies
6. CFS is Vitamin Deficiencies or Imbalances
7. CFS is Mineral Deficiencies or Imbalances
8. CFS is Amino Acid Deficiencies or Imbalances
9. CFS is Enzyme Deficiencies of Imbalances
10. CFS is Sjögren's Syndrome
11. CFS is Essential Fatty Acid Deficiencies or Imbalances
12. CFS is Celiac Disease
13. CFS is Malnutrition
14. CFS is Slow Brain Functioning
15. CFS is Fast Brain Functioning

16. CFS is Hypersensitivity to Light
17. CFS is Hypersensitivity to Sound
18. CFS is Hypersensitivity to Odor
19. CFS is Dysrhythmia between Breathing and Heart Rate
20. CFS is Pointed-Head Syndrome
21. CFS is Mycoplasma (Fermentans) (Incognitus)
22. CFS is Flukes
23. CFS is Epstein-Barr Virus
24. CFS is Cytomegalic Virus
25. CFS is Herpes Virus
26. CFS is Post-Polio Malaise
27. CFS is Thyroid Dysfunction
28. CFS is Sleep Apnea
29. CFS is Hypothyroidism
30. CFS is Pituitary Dysfunction
31. CFS is Hypothymus Dysfunction
32. CFS is Adrenal Exhaustion
33. CFS is Kidney Dysfunction
34. CFS is Liver Toxicity
35. CFS is Mitochondria Dysfunction
36. CFS is Hypoglycemia
37. CFS is Insulin Resistance

38. CFS is Diabetes
39. CFS is Whiplash
40. CFS is Slipped Disc
41. CFS is Pinched Nerve
42. CFS is Emotional Trauma
43. CFS is Post Traumatic Stress Disorder
44. CFS is Spiritual Trauma
45. CFS is Attention Deficit Disorder
46. CFS is Attention Deficit Hyperactivity Disorder
47. CFS is not Lupus
48. CFS is not Lyme disease
49. CFS is not anything else
50. CFS is Fibromyalgia but with much less pain

These are the most important things I believe that cause CFS. I say this after interviewing hundreds of people with CFS and from my own personal experiences.

I spoke with hundreds of patients at various clinics I attended as well as so many of the 400 members of the Chronic Fatigue Syndrome and Fibromyalgia Research and Support Group of San Diego, California, which Ms. Jo Nost and I co-chaired for about five years in the late 1990's. Most of our members had CFS or Fibromyalgia, but a few were our supporters and caregivers.

Obviously, my conversations were not scientific, but they gave me a good understanding about the recurring causes and problems associated with CFS and Fibromyalgia.

14

Fibromyalgia Is
The Same as CFS
But with Limited Fatigue

After listening to hundreds of people with CFS and Fibromyalgia, I have seen and heard how similar these two illnesses are. I consider Fibromyalgia to be the sister illness of CFS.

People with Fibromyalgia have many of the same symptoms and problems as people with CFS, but they have less or little fatigue or exhaustion. CFS emphasizes the fatigue and exhaustion while Fibromyalgia emphasizes the pain.

15

Fibromyalgia Is
A Kidney Disorder Which Causes
Plaque to Accumulate in the Cells

Dr. R. Paul St. Amand, M.D., endocrinologist, Marina Del Rey, Los Angeles, California, believes that almost all Fibromyalgia patients have a kidney disorder, which creates plaque (calcium phosphate) in the cells, and that plaque causes severe pain throughout the body.

Dr. St. Amand's remedy is to use large doses of Guifenisen. Unfortunately, that medication caused me to have excessive constipation, so he prescribed the medication Sulfinpyrazone, which is now available for purchase by prescription from Canada.

His contribution to saving the lives of many people with Fibromyalgia cannot be overestimated. My life has been greatly improved because of his medical discovery. For those so inclined, I suggest viewing his website for more information.

I had a huge success using his protocol, and I thank him immensely for his contributions to this field of medicine, because during much of my life, the plaque caused by muscles to be hard as rock.

But, to be honest, I have known many others who have not been as fortunate as I. For those who have not responded well to his protocol or will not respond well, I have found there are other causes and remedies for Fibromyalgia, which I list and discuss next in this book.

16

Fibromyalgia
Other Causes

1. Flukes: infection and die-off
2. Yeast and Fungus: infection and die-off
3. Mycoplasma: infection and die-off
4. Lyme disease
5. DHEA problems
4. Adrenal exhaustion
5. Post-Polio Syndrome
6. Hypoglycemia
7. Lymph system toxicity
8. Heavy metal toxicity
9. Leaky Gut Syndrome
10. Sleep Apnea
11. Vitamin D Deficiency
12. Vitamin B Deficiencies
13. Mineral Imbalances and Deficiencies
14. Amino acid Imbalances and Deficiencies
15. Essential Fatty Acid Imbalances and Deficiencies
16. Bad mattresses

17. Whiplash
18. Pinched nerves
19. Pointy-head syndrome
20. Damaged Tendons and Ligaments
21. Toxic muscles
21. Damaged Cartilage
22. Stored or Repressed Negative Emotions
23. Post-Traumatic Stress Disorder

17

Prolotherapy Helps
Fibromyalgia Points of Pain

Prolotherapy is the injection of a benign substance into the ligaments and tendons to repair irritated and chronically injured tissue. At *Prolotherapy.com*, the website states:

"Prolotherapy is also known as nonsurgical ligament reconstruction. Prolotherapy uses a dextrose (sugar water) solution, which is injected into the ligament or tendon where it attaches to the bone. This causes a localized inflammation in these weak areas, which then increases the blood supply and flow of nutrients, and stimulates the tissue to repair itself."

18

Chasing and Popping
Fibromyalgia Points of Pain

I discovered a technique that slowly reduced my Fibromyalgia Points of Pain. Literally, I had thousands of them.

When I was lying on the couch or bed, I closed my eyes and located the Worst Fibromyalgia Point of Pain in my body.

Then, I did the following **Technique**:

1. I Squeezed My Muscles Until I Found the Most Painful Fibro Point of Pain in My Body.

2. I Zeroed In On That Specific Fibro Point of Pain.

3. I Relaxed All Other Muscles in My Body.

4. I Squeezed the Fibro Point of Pain As Hard As I Could For As Long As I Could.

5. I Rested

6. I Repeated

7. I Located the Next Most Painful Fibro Point in My Body.

8. I Zeroed In On That One.

9. I Relaxed All Other Muscles.

10. I Squeeze the Muscle With That Fibro Point of Pain As Hard As I Could For As Long As I Could.

11. I Rested.

12. *I REPEATED UNTIL THERE WERE NO MORE FIBRO POINTS OF PAIN, OR UNTIL MY TIME RAN OUT, OR, UNTIL I BECAME TOO EXHAUSTED TO CONTINUE.*

13. **I knew I had reached the "Most Important Fibro Point of Pain," when I had squeezed it for as long as I could, and then, I began to *Fibrillate*.**

14. The **Fibrillation** lasted a few minutes.

19

Repressed or Suppressed Memories
Can Cause Fibro Points of Pain

My Fibro Points of Pain were located in the knots in my muscles. Some of the knots were created by tensions that had started when I was very young.

Sometimes, when I fibrillated, a flashback or memory of some tension-filled incident with some person would come to mind.

I realized that one cause of a Fibro Point of Pain was the tension stored in the core in the knot in the muscle.

I realized that the muscle knotted into a ball of pain because there was a very specific incident of tension.

I realized that the muscle stayed knotted in a ball of pain because the memory was stored in the tension-filled muscle.

I realized that when I squeezed that last Worst Fibro Point of Pain as hard as I could for as long as I could, and then fibrillated, the flashback appeared in my memory and then disappeared.

At the same time, the knot in my muscle and the Fibro Point of Pain dissolved and disappeared. Both were gone forever.

I realized that this flashback of memory and the dissolution and disappearance process of the knot in my muscle and the Fibro Point of Pain occurred only when I fibrillated.

Each time it happened, it was a very exhausting process, but it left me exhilarated. *It also left me with much less pain.*

Popping and dissolving the Fibro Points of Pain was a very fascinating, exhilarating, long-term process.

Over time, I removed over 99.9% of the Fibro Points of Pain from my body.

I am very happy not to have them anymore.

20

Chasing and Popping Fibro Points of Pain
The Technique in Plain English

I started by lying down in a comfortable position, usually on my bed, and then I closed my eyes.

I started by squeezing all my muscles and discovered which Fibro Point of Pain was the worst.

I squeezed the muscle that contained the *Worst* Fibro Point of Pain. I squeezed that muscle as hard as I could for as long as I could.

Then, I gradually focused on the specific Fibro Point of Pain.

I squeezed that Fibro Point of Pain as hard as I could for as long as I could.

Then, I rested.

Then, I repeated.

I would find and locate the Next Worst Fibro Point of Pain and repeat the process.

I literally chased the Fibro Points of Pain around my body for an hour or two each day.

After an hour or two, there came a time when there was no worst Fibro Point of Pain.

After I squeezed the Last Worst Fibro Point of Pain for the day, as hard as I could for as long as I could, I began to **Fibrillate**!

My body shook for a minute or two.

Then, I knew I had popped a major center of tension and pain. Many times a repressed memory or flashback popped up.

If that happened, it was an image of a person with whom I had had some previous tension.

I knew that the tension had been stored in a knot in my muscle, and it was causing a Fibro Point of Pain.

By squeezing that Fibro Point of Pain as hard as I could for as long as I could, I released the memory that was causing the muscle to stay knotted.

After that knot was released, that Fibro Point of Pain was released too, and both disappeared forever.

I have used this technique for more than three years. It has eliminated over 99.9% of my Fibro Points of Pain.

I am now virtually free from Fibro Points of Pain.

Hallelujah!

In Conclusion

For those who wish to know my present status, at almost 65 years of age, I am left with some minor pains, which appear if I work or exercise too hard, become too stressed out, or the weather changes.

The level of **pain that I now have is hardly noticeable** compared to the level of pain I lived with for decades.

To say the least,

I am one very happy camper!

21

Medical Cannabis (Marijuana)
May Reduce or Eliminate
CFS and Fibromyalgia Pain

When I am have exercised too much, worked too hard, have felt too much stress, or the weather changes, I feel some residual CFS exhaustion or some minor residual Fibromyalgia pain.

I found that a little good quality medical cannabis (marijuana) reduces or eliminates my residual CFS and Fibromyalgia as well as some minor depression. A good sativa elevates my mood and makes me happy!

For occasional pain, I still use a little gabapentin (Neurontin) or an over-the-counter pain reliever.

I find exercise of no value for relieving my CFS or Fibromyalgia. In fact, exercise makes my pain worse if I do it more than I can safely handle.

The amount of exercise I can tolerate varies. It depends upon my mood, the level of my vitality, the level of my physical strength and my inner joy.

I do not exercise beyond my capabilities because **if I do too much, I will suffer** a significant *increase* in *pain* and *exhaustion* for a period of time.

Obviously, an increase in those negative side effects is not good and to be avoided!

22

Silver/Mercury Fillings
Can Cause CFS and Fibromyalgia

The fillings in my teeth were made mostly of *silver* and *mercury*. The *mercury* in those fillings caused:

(1) Yeast and Fungus Overgrowth, which caused:

(2) Leaky Gut Syndrome, which caused:

(3) Allergies, hives and psoriasis,

(4) CFS, Fibromyalgia, Depression, Brain Fog, Confusion, Central Nervous System Dysfunction, Balance Problems.

For almost a century, in the U.S., dental fillings were made by mixing a few metals together according the following general formula.

25% silver,

50% mercury,

12% zinc, and

3% of a few other metals

One of my medical professional consultants poked ironic fun at the American Dental Establishment by saying:

"When *mercury* arrives at the dentist's office, it comes in a container that is clearly marked 'Poison'.

"And, when *mercury* is removed from a patient's mouth, the dentist places it into a container that is clearly marked 'Poison'.

"**But**, while *mercury* is in a patient's mouth, dentists tell patients that 'those fillings are safe and harmless.' *How absurd*!"

It is *not acceptable* for anyone to say that fillings containing mercury are safe and harmless.

23

Methyl Mercury Gas

In addition, **methyl mercury gas** can be produced when someone chews food while they have a silver/mercury filling in their mouth.

Sometimes, the level of methyl mercury in a person's mouth can be over 1,000 times greater than what is legally permitted to be in the environment by the U.S. government.

It is obvious that *some people are poisoning themselves into sickness or early death by the methyl mercury gas that is in their mouths.*

However, we, the people, are *not* informed by our doctors or dentists of this toxic gas or its harmful effects.

It is not unreasonable to believe that many people with CFS, Fibromyalgia and other disorders have become very sick and died from the toxic effects of having silver/**mercury** fillings put into their mouths.

If they had been informed about silver/**mercury** fillings' toxicity, many people would have been spared much misery.

The **good** news is that for most people it appears that when mercury breaks off from a filling, it is excreted by the body without causing too much harm.

Also, it appears that for most people, they do not suffer too much from methyl mercury toxicity.

The **bad** news is that many CFS patients and Fibromyalgia patients are absorbers of heavy metals, **including mercury**, and *we are badly affected by mercury and methyl mercury gas.*

24

Mercury Causes "Leaky Gut Syndrome"

Mercury acts as an antibiotic. It kills both good and bad bacteria. When it kills good bacteria in the colon, yeast can grow beyond its normal, healthy limit. Then, yeast is able to change into fungus, and yeast and fungus multiply into the danger zone.

Fungus is very dangerous because it is able to drill holes through the walls of the colon and then enter into the bloodstream. It literally creates holes in the colon.

Holes in the colon allow yeast, fungus, pathogens and unnatural proteins to pass into the bloodstream from the colon. Those things were supposed to stay in the colon and not get into the bloodstream.

When yeast, fungus, pathogens or unnatural proteins enter the bloodstream, each can trigger the immune system to react a lot. A severe immune system reaction can cause the patient to experience mild to severe allergy attacks, hives, psoriasis, auto-immune disorders, or feel like he or she is always experiencing the flu or a chronic infection.

When a patient experiences the discomfort, pain, fatigue and suffering of having holes in his or her colon or of having unnatural things pass through them, he or she is said to be suffering from **"Leaky Gut Syndrome."**

In addition, while in the bloodstream, yeast and fungus are being attacked by the immune system. Their death causes *die-off.* **Die-off can cause severe reactions.** *Die-off* can cause mild to severe allergic reactions, hives, psoriasis, fatigue, exhaustion, cognition problems and mild to severe abdominal bloating. These are also symptoms of the "Leaky Gut Syndrome."

Yeast and fungal infections in the bloodstream, can affect the brain. If the brain is affected, the patient can suffer various mental and physical illnesses, *including depression, cognitive challenges, confusion, brain fog, short-term memory loss, and balance problems.*

Please note that because the above illnesses were caused by yeast and fungal infections that affected my brain, medications such as **Diflucan** and **Sporanox** have helped me (and others) **recover** from these problems.

Leaky Gut Syndrome can be remedied with **butyric acid** treatment. Butyric acid is a component of butter and ghee. It helps the body close the holes created by fungus.

Once the holes are repaired, the yeast, fungus and other pathogens and proteins will no longer be able to reach the bloodstream, and the symptoms of Leaky Gut Syndrome will diminish or subside completely.

Afterwards, glutathione, yeast and fungal killers, and probiotics can be used to help reduce and heal the problems associated with Leaky Gut Syndrome.

25

Lead Can Cause
CFS and Fibromyalgia

Lead is a very toxic heavy metal. It has been proven that it can cause major neurological disorders, especially in children.

Lead poisoning leaves you feeling very tired, exhausted, mentally dull and achy. It causes CFS and Fibromyalgia.

The U.S. government has a policy of wanting to prevent people, especially children, from developing severe neurological disorders caused by consuming lead based paint or breathing lead based gasoline.

Because lead is so dangerous, the U.S. government ordered automobile manufacturing companies to stop producing cars that use leaded gasoline and produce automobiles that use unleaded gasoline.

Because lead is so damaging to the brain, the U.S. government ordered gasoline manufacturers and paint makers to remove it from production in 1979.

Unfortunately for me, I stored large amounts of lead. As a result, I ended up with significant neurological disorders, which caused extreme exhaustion, memory problems, cognition and balance difficulties.

I believe that because I had celiac disease, my body stored lead instead of excreting it.

On a daily basis, for decades, unknown to me, I was being poisoned by lead and other heavy metals, *until I* removed them by using colonics.

26

Where I Was Exposed to Lead

Some places where I was exposed to and ingested lead:

(1) I ate the paint off of the No. 2 orange pencils I used in elementary school.

(2) I smelled and inhaled leaded gasoline.

(3) I drank tap water which contained lead. Lead was leached into the water from the solder that was used to weld the copper water pipes together.

(4) I ate lead-based paint which was on the slats off my baby crib.

(5) I breathed and inhaled first hand and second hand cigarette smoke.

27

Regulation of Heavy Metals
Is Good Business

Environmental regulation is **necessary for personal safety**, but it is also **very good for business.**

When you consider how many *millions* of people are *disabled* partially or fully, mentally or physically, because they suffer from heavy metal poisoning, **lost productivity and payments to the disabled make the costs of heavy metal toxicity staggering**.

Protecting people from heavy metal poisoning is not just **doing good** for people, but it is also **doing good for business.**

28

A Badly Functioning Immune System
Can Cause CFS and Fibromyalgia

When the immune system is very active, you feel very sick and tired. You feel like you have the flu.

If you have "Leaky Gut Syndrome," chronic infections or chronic parasite infestations, your immune system will be very active all the time. Then you will feel very sick and tired *all the time*.

The immune system stays active when it is trying to kill the invading bugs but it is not able to kill all of them. It must stay active in order to stop them from growing, proliferating and eventually killing your body.

The immune system stays active all the time when it has sufficient numbers of white blood cells to fight the bugs, but those white blood cells are not strong enough to kill all of the bugs. Then the immune system will be active all the time.

When that happens, you will feel sick and tired, exhausted with aches and pain *all the time.*

When that happens, life will become very grim.

If that happens, you can become chronically depressed.

29

A Dysfunctional Part
of the Immune System
Can Cause CFS and Fibromyalgia

When you do not have a certain part of your immune system, the bugs, germs, and pathogens can multiply.

You will feel sick and tired when the bugs take over your body.

You will feel sick and tired when they emit a lot of their waste.

You will feel sick and tired when they die-off.

There are many different parts to the immune system. If any of the parts are not functioning well or is missing, your body may not be able to rid itself of the invading germs. If that happens you will feel sick and tired and in pain *all the time*.

There are immune system specialists who have tests to determine the state of your immune system.

There are medicines to improve and repair a dysfunctional immune system.

It is important to know that CFS and Fibromyalgia can be caused by one or more problems with one or more parts of your immune system.

30

Celiac Disease and Malnutrition Can Cause CFS

Celiac disease has been diagnosed for about 1% of the U.S. population. That means about 3.3 million people in the U.S. have the disease.

Millions of Americans should not be eating wheat, oats, rye or barley, and products which contain those grains.

Eating those grains causes problems both large and small to people who have celiac disease.

Earlier I wrote about how celiac disease caused me to:

1. suffer severe constipation starting when I was a young child,

2. stunted my growth as an older child,

3. blocked elimination as an adult, which forced me to go the Emergency Room for treatment of my severe abdominal pain,

4. led to storing heavy metals until I was poisoned by them, and

5. made suicidal.

Celiac disease also caused me to suffer severe malabsorption. It prevented enough nutrients from being absorbed by my body to cause severe fatigue and exhaustion (CFS).

When I did not absorb sufficient nutrients, such as Vitamin D3, I felt very tired, to the point of feeling exhausted and kind of suicidal.

To increase my energy, I have used one or all of the following separately or together as needed:

A 50 mg. of vitamin B complex
A general amino acid complex
A vitamin D3 capsule

To better digest *and* absorb nutrients *from my food, I use a* general herbal enzyme supplement.

31

Celiac Disease and
A Low Carbohydrate Diet

Eating a low carbohydrate diet to lose weight may work for some people because they have celiac disease.

If someone has celiac disease and **stops eating wheat** and other grains which contain the harmful gluten, **their body will stop retaining fluids and start eliminating more waste and fluids.**

As a result, they will lose weight and size.

I think this is a reasonable explanation simply because it happened to me.

32

Slow Brain Functioning
Can Cause CFS and Fibromyalgia

Many people have had brain injuries from whiplash or concussions. Those traumas may have *slowed* the functioning of their brains so that their brains are partially asleep despite the fact that they are awake.

This feels like they are tired all the time, mentally sluggish and confused. Memory problems are triggered by slow brain functioning, too.

Fibromyalgia may be caused by slow brain functioning as well.

33

Fast Brain Functioning
Can Cause CFS and Fibromyalgia

Many people have had brain injuries from whiplash or concussions. These traumas may have *increased* the functioning of their brains so their brains do not rest while asleep. This can lead to total exhaustion. They are tired and in pain all the time. I have used Neurontin (gabapentin) to help resolve this problem.

Beware, gabapentin can become a trap. I have known a few people who started using this medicine but had trouble stopping it when it was not effective or it was no longer effective.

Considering the challenges some people have had with this medicine, it is probably best to use the lowest dose possible, because it can become great trouble if you have to stop using it.

34

Hypersensitivity to Light
May Cause CFS

Those who are hypersensitive to light may become very tired. Eye drops may help alleviate this problem.

35

Hypersensitivity to Sound
and Odor May Cause CFS

Excessive sounds or odors may cause or be caused by CFS or Fibromyalgia.

Sometimes hypersensitivity to sound and odor may be caused by low vitality of the immune system or mitochondria.

I have increased vitamins, minerals, amino acids, essential fatty acids, enzymes, **sunshine,** mild exercise, gentle breathing exercises, meditating, and reducing stress to increase vitality levels.

I use Lamictal (lamotrigine) to reduce my hypersensitivities to light, sound and odors.

Excessive light, sound and odors can cause allergic reactions. Benedryl and other anti-allergy medications may be beneficial to stop excessive reactions by the body to light, sound and odors.

36

Dysrhythmia between Breathing
and the Heart Rate May Cause CFS

One graduate student in psychology researched the relationship between the breathing rate and the heart rate in CFS patients.

He told me that preliminary results showed that:

In healthy individuals, the breathing rate and heart rate were synchronized. But, in CFS patients, that was not true.

The theory is too new to evaluate, but it could be something to think about in the future.

37

Pointed Head Syndrome
May Cause CFS and Fibromyalgia

Some babies come from the womb with the top bones of their head forming a ridge. If not corrected, those bones will continue to grow that way into adulthood, and they will form a pointed ridge down the top of the head on the adult. Since the ridge is covered over with hair. it generally goes unnoticed later in life.

However, some healers believe that having a bony head ridge has negative effects on health which can lead to CFS or Fibromyalgia.

The theory is: If the bones are interlocked, they will not expand and contract as intended while breathing. Failure to do so may lead to toxicity, fatigue and pain, because the spinal-cerebral pump is not fully activated.

It is something to consider because I have been told by some healers that some people have had great relief by removing the pointed ridge on their heads through therapy (not surgery).

Personally, I used constant head, neck and trapezius massage plus moderate pushing on my head bones to move them into their normal position. It took about three years from the time I was 48 to 51 years old, but now I have a round head without a pointed head or ridge running down the center of my skull.

38

Flukes Can Cause
CFS and Fibromyalgia

Flukes are flat worms that may come from eating meat. They are parasites which can cause fatigue and pain, CFS and Fibromyalgia.

39

Epstein - Barr Virus
Can Cause CFS and Fibromyalgia

EBV is a herpes virus. If it is not suppressed by the immune system, it can cause continuous exhaustion. If not totally suppressed by the immune system, it can cause unremitting activation of the immune system. An over-active immune system can cause CFS and Fibromyalgia.

EBV is contagious, usually transmitted by kissing. It is commonly known as mononucleosis.

It is not considered a primary cause of CFS or Fibromyalgia because people recover from it on a regular basis, and it is its own disease.

40

Cytomegalic Virus Can
Cause CFS and Fibromyalgia

Cytomegalic virus, if not suppressed by the immune system, can cause continuous exhaustion and pain, thus causing CFS and Fibromyalgia.

Like any other constant viral infection that is not destroyed or suppressed, the virus may cause CFS and Fibromyalgia.

As discussed before, a constantly activated immune system, which is trying to destroy the CMV, can cause CFS and Fibromyalgia.

41

Herpes Viruses Can Cause CFS and Fibromyalgia

There are many herpes viruses. If any are not suppressed by the immune system, they can cause continuous exhaustion and pain. They may cause unremitting activation of the immune system. That, too, can cause CFS and Fibromyalgia.

42

Post-Polio Malaise
and Adrenal Exhaustion
Can Cause CFS and Fibromyalgia

CFS and Fibromyalgia patients who exercise too much may suffer exhaustion for days or weeks afterwards.

CFS exhaustion is similar to what polio victims suffer after they exercise too much. That condition is called Post-Polio Malaise.

*For CFS and Fibromyalgia patients, I believe that **adrenal exhaustion** and **DHEA** deficiency problems play large roles, especially when there are significant post exercise malaise problems.*

43

Sleep Apnea Can Cause
CFS and Fibromyalgia

Sleep apnea is a neurological disorder that prevents patients from getting sleep that fully rejuvenates the body, mind and spirit.

As a result of not getting fully rejuvenating sleep, patients suffer chronic exhaustion like those who suffer from CFS and Fibromyalgia.

You can have sleep apnea, CFS and Fibromyalgia together. They are not mutually exclusive.

44

Hypothyroidism Can Cause CFS, Fibromyalgia, Confusion, and Depression

Hypothyroidism is a medical condition where the thyroid gland is not performing well. As a result, the body's internal temperature is cold. The hair is brittle and lusterless. The patient will feel sluggish and depressed, too. Aches and pains are felt as well.

Doctors do not treat borderline hypothyroidism because they generally do not believe that a cold body is too important. They are taught to believe that a hot body, one that has a fever, is in danger from infection or disease, and thus, is in need of immediate treatment.

They are taught that a cold body is not in great danger of dying or becoming very ill very soon, so that problem is not in urgent need of treatment.

Nevertheless, it is a *big* problem for those of us who live in bodies that are chronically under-performing.

For example, think of an automobile. It is designed to work best at a certain temperature. If it is constantly running cold, the mechanic will try to discover what is wrong and fix the problem in order to **maximize performance**.

However, doctors do not think like mechanics. They are too worried about life threatening illnesses to be very concerned about people who are struggling through the day because their bodies are under-performing.

However, it is very important to have an internal body temperature that is within the normal functioning range. Otherwise, all other bodily systems will *not* function well, either.

The normal internal temperature for best functioning is around 98.6° Fahrenheit.

If you **feel cold** or have other symptoms of hypothyroidism, you may be a candidate for treatment. You may respond very well to supplemental treatments.

Lastly: For those who **suffer from cold feet at night,** *I found that I had to **bundle up** to cure my cold feet!*

I use a shirt, an undershirt, and a hoodie to keep my upper body and head warm. *When I keep my upper body and head warm, my lower body, feet and toes stay very nice and warm, too.*

All of this helps me sleep better at night. I wake up feeling more refreshed, relaxed and happier.

45

Gulf War Syndrome
May Be Caused By
Mycoplasma Fermentans Incognitus

Mycoplasma fermentans incognitus causes CFS, Fibromyalgia, depression, rage and *may be the primary cause of Gulf War Syndrome.*

Mycoplasma is its own kind of bug. It's a pathogen that is sort of like yeast and sort of like bacteria.

If you become infected by *mycoplasma, it is very hard to get rid of.* It is very contagious. It can be given to animals as well. It causes fatigue, exhaustion, pain, confusion, memory problems, rage, anger and brain fog.

Mycoplasma fermentans incognitus is a very specific type of mycoplasma that is even harder to get rid of than normal.

It was created and patented (No. 5,242,820) by a scientist working for the U.S. government as a Biological Weapon of Mass Destruction. It was created as a vehicle for *warfare.* It was created to infect the enemy and cause total disability, but not death.

It was meant to debilitate many soldiers and support staff and civilians, but not kill them. It was meant to cause the enemy to use huge amounts of manpower, energy and supplies to take care of their sick, and thus hinder their ability to wage war effectively.

It is thought to be *the **primary cause** of the Gulf War Syndrome* by Dr. Garth Nicolson, Ph.D. who testified to this fact before Congress.

46

How I Killed Mycoplasma

I have had two major infections of mycoplasma in the past twenty years. It is unknown whether it grew back after a decade's relapse, or I contracted it a second time from another source.

Here are the different two ways I killed it.

(A) To kill *mycoplasma* recently (in 2012), I used **colloidal silver injections** three times a week for 8 months to a year.

(B) To kill *mycoplasma fermentans incognitus* more than ten years ago, I used a **combination of therapies**.

First, I saturated my body with oxygen at 10 liters of pressure for two hours twice per day by breathing it through a face.

I did this because oxygen weakens this parasite.

I believe that using a hyperbaric chamber to saturate the body with oxygen would also work well to weaken this parasite.

Second, I used the antibiotic Doxycycline.

Third, I used an immune system booster called, Transfer Factor, which was prepared by Dr. Said Youdim, Ph.D. of Los Angeles, California.

Fourth, I used an anti-allergy substance prepared at the clinic owned by Dr. William Ray in Dallas, Texas.

Fifth, I used my mind to create an environment that was inhospitable to the parasite.

Every day, I said to myself that my body was too hot for the mycoplasma to live in and it had to go.

I thought of the following example:

When I think I am sucking on a lemon, my body reacts as if I am actually sucking on a lemon.

I realized if I thought that my body was too hot for the parasite to survive in, it will become too hot for the mycoplasma to survive in. Thus, it will have to leave or die.

Every day, I told my body to make it impossible for the mycoplasma to live in.

Every day I told my body that the mycoplasma had to leave.

Every day, I told the mycoplasma it had to go.

Sixth, I put a low grade electrical current on my body to change my body's electrical frequency. This made my body's electrical frequency inhospitable to the mycoplasma.

The electricity generator was sold by Dr. Hulda Clark of San Diego, California. Now, the company is called "Clarkia."

Seventh, I prayed and had others pray for me.

Eighth, Ozone Therapy may also destroy mycoplasma.

47

Obesity
and Toxicity

When I first removed the heavy metals by using colonics, I lost a lot of weight and size quickly and easily.

I believe that *my fat cells stored the heavy metals because my body was not able to safely dispose of them during normal bowel movements or when urinating.*

When my fat cells were storing the heavy metals, dieting did not work for me. Once the heavy metals were being safely removed from my fat cells, I was able to lose a lot of weight and size quickly.

As the heavy metals were being removed, I lost about 40 lbs. I went from 245 to 205 lbs., and I have maintained that weight for more than 15 years.

48

Obesity and Essential Fatty Acids

Olive oil, flax oil, borage oil, fish oil, CLA and Evening Primrose oil may be necessary in various amounts for some people to balance their diets and stop binge eating.

Each oil contains different properties. Some may reduce depression, which may be a cause of binge eating.

I found **Evening Primrose oil**, which is well known for reducing mood disorders, including **pre-menstrual syndrome**, to be an effective mood elevator for me. It seems **to help** *relieve my depression*.

However, it did not help me lose weight. But, it may help some people.

49

Obesity Can Be Caused
By Yeast and Fungus

I have observed that when I was suffering from too much yeast and fungus in my body, I became bloated and heavier. But, when I took **Diflucan** or **Sporanox** for a few days, I became less bloated and lost weight.

Why? Did my fat cells retain fluids as a defense against being invaded by yeast and fungus? Did my cells retain fluids to ward off the yeast and fungus invading them?

I do not know the answer to these questions. However, it is interesting to note that:

Whenever I stopped eating sugar, bread, or starch, and I stopped drinking alcohol --- all things which yeast and fungus love --- I did not become bloated, and I lost weight.

Others have reported the same thing to me, so I am sure there must be a **connection** between yeast, fungus, bloating and obesity.

50

Obesity and Yeast

Yeast loves sugar, bread, starch and alcohol.

Once yeast starts to feed on these things, it grows and demands more.

Once it grows and enters the bloodstream, it eats the sugar that was meant to nourish the brain.

Since sugar is the primary source of energy for the brain, not enough sugar in the bloodstream is a major problem for the body and brain. Without enough sugar, the brain will not work very well, and the body will become jittery and faint. That is the essence of *hypoglycemia.*

The brain demands sugar to function. It demands to be fed very fast. Otherwise, it and the body will not survive.

Without enough sugar, you feel jittery, faint, aggressive or exhausted. Those symptoms are known as having the "sugar blues."

When we need sugar fast, we reach for sugar, bread, starch or alcohol. Each of those things are converted into sugar and can be used by the brain very fast.

This process floods the bloodstream with sugar, and feeds the brain. *It also feeds the yeast.* And this process also makes us fatter.

As we feed the brain, we feed the yeast. The brain is fed but so is the yeast. The more we feed the brain, the more the yeast grows.

As the yeast grows, it demands more food. It eats the sugar that the brain needs. Thus, the brain is deprived of the sugar it needs. The brain screams for more sugar. We get the sugar blues. We feed it sugar. We feed the brain. We feed the yeast. That process results is known as *hypoglycemia.*

And, as we eat more sugar, bread, starch and alcohol, we grow fatter.

Because of yeast, we eat too much of things like ice cream, potato chips, French fries, ketchup, and drink too much soda pop and alcohol. Literally, as we feed our brains, we grow our yeast.

**Yum for Us, and
Yum for Our Yeast ---
As We Grow
More Obese.**

51

Alcoholism Can Be
Caused By Yeast and Fungus

Yeast loves sugar, bread, starch and ALCOHOL. Once yeast starts to feed on these items, it grows and demands more.

Once yeast enters the bloodstream, it eats the sugar that was meant to feed the brain.

Since sugar is the primary source of energy for the brain, the lack of sugar in the bloodstream is a major problem for the brain. When there is too little sugar in the bloodstream, the brain demands to be fed more sugar --- fast.

As a result, we feed the brain sugar, bread, starch or ALCOHOL, all of which are converted into sugar for the brain very fast.

This process floods the bloodstream with sugar, which feeds the brain, but, it feeds the yeast and fungus as well.

The result is that your brain is happy, the yeast and fungus are happy, and we grow fatter.

When we Feed the Brain,
We Feed the Yeast and Fungus.
The brain is fed, but
So are the yeast and fungus.
The more we feed the brain,
The bigger the yeast and fungus grow.

This Is A Vicious Cycle.
This Is the Yeast Monster.

As the yeast grows, it demands more sugar, bread, starch, or ALCOHOL.

Some people's brains crave ALCOHOL. If that happens, they suffer from *Alcoholism.*

The more ALCOHOL they drink, the more they feed their yeast and fungus.

As their yeast and fungus grow, they deprive their brains of sugar.

Then their brains demand that they feed it more ALCOHOL.

Repeat.

Hence, they become ALCOHOLICS.

Drink ALCOHOL!
Yum for them, and
Yum for their yeast and fungus.

At an Alcoholics Anonymous meeting, the participants eat lots of DONUTS AND COOKIES, and drink coffee with lots of SUGAR AND MILK.

Obviously, Alcoholics are:

SUBSTITUTING
SUGAR, BREAD
AND STARCH for ALCOHOL.
THEY DO THIS TO FEED THEIR YEAST.

In my opinion, if *Alcoholics would reduce their yeast and fungus*, they would *be able to reduce their alcoholism* as well.

From my observations, this makes perfectly good sense to me.

52

Foul Smelling Feces Can Cause CFS, Fibromyalgia, Confusion and Depression

Foul Smelling Feces (FSF) is human waste matter which has been stored in the colon and small intestine for a long time. It can cause CFS, Fibromyalgia, Confusion, Depression, Obesity, Alcoholism and Death.

Foul Smelling Feces is human waste matter that has been partly digested and left putrefying in the body. It creates **flatulence** and foul smelling feces.

Rotting, putrefying waste matter in the colon and small intestine transmits toxins and breeds pathogens.

Those things can cause CFS, Fibromyalgia, chronic depression, confusion, brain fog, chronic illness, aches, pains and even early death.

The idea that storing rotting, putrefying waste matter in the body is a leading cause of many illnesses is not readily understood by many medical doctors and other health practitioners.

Dr. Bernard Jensen, Ph.D., N.D., did some amazing, ground-breaking work in this area.

His book, **"Tissue Cleansing through Bowel Management,"** should be read and studied by all persons who are seriously interested in healthy living and recovery.

53

Foul Smelling Feces
Can Cause Obesity

Rotting, putrefying waste matter which is being stored in the body is a prime breeding ground for toxic pathogens, such as excessive amounts of yeast and fungus. After these pathogens work themselves from the colon into the bloodstream, they can attack cells.

One defense used by cells against attack from pathogens is to become more rigid. They do this by retaining fluids. Like a balloon that retains water, retaining liquid makes the outer membrane of the cell harder and thus less susceptible to invasion. However, *when the body retains fluids, it becomes heavier and obese.*

When the putrefying waste matter is removed from the colon and small intestine, yeast and fungus are reduced.

Then, the cells retain less fluid.

As a result, the body loses weight and reduces size.

54

Foul Smelling Feces
Can Cause Alcoholism

Rotting, putrefying waste matter stored in the body is a breeding ground for pathogens, such as excessive yeast and fungus.

As the yeast and fungus work themselves from the colon into the bloodstream, they attack the cells, organs and affect the brain. They attack and destroy sugar, which the brain needs to survive.

Some people who have an overload of fungus and yeast in their bodies have brains that demand that they use alcohol as the primary source of food for their yeast, fungus and brain. They are called, **Alcoholics**.

If those people removed the Foul Smelling Feces, which is the putrefying waste matter in their colons, they would also reduce the breeding ground for excessive yeast and fungus in their bodies, which causes them to crave alcohol.

For alcoholics, if they eliminated FSF, yeast and fungus would be reduced. The result would be that their cravings for alcohol would be reduced, as well.

55

Antibiotics Can Help
Chronic Viral Infections

Antibiotics kill bacteria. They do not kill viruses or infections caused by viruses. So, doctors do not prescribe antibiotics for killing viral infections.

However, antibiotics may play a role in reducing viral infections. If there are many infections, including viral and bacterial infections, using antibiotics will reduce the amount of bacterial infections that the immune system must fight.

A reduction in the level of bacterial infections will increase the amount of energy available for the immune system to use to fight viral infections.

For those people who have an immune system that is not strong enough to kill enough viruses, it may be necessary to use antibiotics against their bacterial infections *in order to free up more energy so that that energy can be used* in the body's fight against their stubborn, overwhelming viral infections.

56

Sometimes Antibiotics
Help Rheumatoid Arthritis

Many years ago, I met a nice older woman who was about 80 years old. She told me that she had suffered from severe rheumatoid arthritis in her hands for decades.

Her disease had become so bad she said that she could not use her hands to open doors by turning doorknobs. Instead, she said, she had to use her elbows.

Her condition had become so intolerable, she said, that she had to seek help from a doctor in another country. He prescribed low doses of an antibiotic three days per week for three months.

As a result of that treatment, she showed me that she could use her hands to open doors by turning doorknobs.

I relay this story for those people who are victims of severe rheumatoid arthritis and who have found nothing else that works to remedy their illness.

57

Tests My Doctors Performed On Me

1.   "Interro" - A Computer Generated Testing Program
2.   Hair Test for Heavy Metals
3.   Hair Test for Mineral Imbalances
4.   Live Blood Cell Test
5.   Mercury Vapor Mouth Test
6.   Mercury Filling Charge Test
7.   Heavy Metal Absorption Test Using a Chelating Provocative Agent
8.   Pesticide Absorption Test
9.   Poisoning from DDT and DDP
10. Poisoning from Propyl Alcohol
11. Poisoning from Benzene
12. Poisoning from Chlorine
13. Poisoning from Fluoride
14. Essential Fatty Acid Absorption and Imbalance Tests
15. Omega 3 and Omega 6 Absorption Tests
16. Free Radical Indication Test

17. Mycoplasma Tests
18. Mycoplasma Fermentans Incognitus
19. Giardia
20. Worms
21. Flukes and Flat Worms
22. Round Worms
23. Pin Worms
24. Yeast
25. Candida
26. Fungus
27. STD's
28. HIV
29. Tuberculosis
30. Acidophilus
31. Vitamin D3 Deficiency
32. Gut Dysbiosis
33. Herpes
34. HHV-6
35. CMV
36. EBV
37. HPV
38. Lyme Disease
39. Cancer
40. Celiac disease

41. Liver Creatine Clearing Test
42. Lymph System Tests
43. Colon Tests
44. Digestion Time Clearance Test
45. Hydrochloric Acid Test
46. Immune System Test of NK Cells
47. Immune System Test, Interleukins 6 and 10 Tests
48. Tumor Necrosis Factor Test
49. Brain Damage using MRI and MRS Tests
50. Thyroid Tests – RTH, TSH
51. Pituitary Tests – HGH
52. Testosterone Test
53. Estrogen Test
54. Adrenal Test
55. Adrenal Stress Index Test
56. Pancreatic Enzyme
57. Urine pH
58. Saliva pH
59. Feces pH
60. Structural Imbalance Tests
61. Uneven Weight Distribution
62. Cranial Misalignment

63. Spinal Misalignment
64. Teeth Balancing
65. Neurological Testing
66. Leaky Gut Test
67. Hypoglycemia Test
68. Fibromyalgia from
    Dr. R. Paul St. Amand
69. Asthma
70. Allergies
71. All Vitamins
72. All Minerals
73. All Amino Acids
74. Standard Testing
75. Sjögren's Syndrome

58

My Basic
Roadmap to Recovery

(1)   Remove Heavy Metals

(2)   Remove Toxic Pesticides and
       Herbicides

(3)   Remove Toxic Waste Matter

(4)   Build up the Immune System

(5)   Reduce or Eliminate Pathogens,
       such as: --- yeast, fungus, mycoplasma,
       worms, flukes, bacteria and viruses

(6)   Repair and Rebuild Organs, Tissues
       and Cells, *such as*:
       Liver, intestines, stomach, adrenals,
       kidneys, thyroid, pituitary,
       hypothalamus, pancreas and lungs

(7)   Repair the Brain

(8)   Repair the Gut

(9)   Reduce Allergies

(10) Reduce Asthma

(11) Reduce Post Traumatic Stress Disorder

(12) Help Others

(13) Surrender to Higher Power

59

Stay Empowered
in the Healing Process

I have been very lucky. I had the money and loving support from a devoted wife so I could go to many caring doctors, healers, dentists, naturopaths, and educated laypersons who guided me back from death's doorstep to life. 21 years later, I am a much healthier, wiser, older man.

Twenty-one years ago, at the end of 1991, I was sleeping 20 hours a day, in constant pain and in constant despair.

Now, I sing, travel, write, ride a motorcycle, help others and scuba dive. My transformation from being totally ill to returning to life has astounded my friends, my family and myself.

The information in this book was gathered in so many ways from those who were so generous with their time, energy, knowledge and wisdom during my recovery.

While I was traveling upon my "Road to Recovery," I learned some important lessons about the human body and the practice of medicine.

Some of the lessons I learned about being a patient in the U.S. were:

Regarding Remedies:
Everything works for somebody, but *not* everything works for everybody.

We are all different. We are all unique.

We all have a lot in common, but we all have a lot of differences.

My doctors and healers were my *consultants*. They did not live in my body.

They saw me for only a brief period of time.

They had thousands of other patients to think about.

I learned that *they could only make* **quick** *and* **educated guesses** *about my health issues.*

I learned that *I should* **not expect** *them to know a lot about me.*

I learned that *I could* **not rely** *exclusively on their judgments.*

I learned that *if I had doubts or I thought something was not going well, it was* **up to me** *to be more assertive.*

I learned that ***I had to make the final decision** about my health care* because it was my body, ***not*** theirs.

I learned that *I had **to take responsibility** for doing what I felt was right for me* because it was my body, not theirs.

I learned that *if something was not going right, then I had **to make a change***.

I learned that *I had to **take charge** of my healthcare*.

I learned that *I had **to be proactive** in my healthcare decisions*.

I learned *I had **to ask questions**,* such as:

"What are the side effects?"
"When should I expect to see results?"

I learned that *if a treatment wasn't working in a reasonable time, then it was time to **try something else***.

I learned that *I had to* **make my life an adventure**, *and regaining my health a challenge.*

I learned that the worst part of being sick in America is that our medical insurance system does **not provide enough money** for all of the things I wanted to do.

I learned that **medical insurance is a very large problem** for most people with our illnesses.

Hopefully, this book will spur Congress and insurance companies to provide additional funding so doctors and healers can provide better testing and treatments for persons with these illnesses.

I learned that:

    it does *not*

        take *much* money

        to get *well*

            once the *causes*

                of these illnesses

                are *found*.

60

About the Author

Marc Herlands graduated from Shaker Heights High School, near Cleveland, Ohio in 1966; Tufts University near Boston, Massachusetts in 1970; Georgetown University Law Center in Washington, D.C. in 1973; and, he earned a Master's degree in tax law from the University of San Diego, California in 1987.

In April 1974, Marc began the practice of law in an eastern suburb of Cleveland, Ohio. In November 1974, at the age of 26, he had his first major attack of Chronic Fatigue Syndrome. By February 1975, he had to stop practicing law full-time because he was so tired, slept poorly, was constantly exhausted, was emotionally upset, depressed, and constantly hungry. His doctor told him he was "burned out," and he had to rest.

From 1975 through 1991, (ages 27 to 43,) Marc passed all of his standard medical tests, but no one could tell him why he was sleeping over 20 hours per day, or why he couldn't sleep without narcotics since his Fibromyalgia pain was so horrible it kept him awake at night.

Beginning in late 1991, his doctor, dentist and other healers began to discover the causes of his health problems. They slowly discovered the causes of his **Chronic Fatigue Syndrome, Fibromyalgia, Gulf War Syndrome, Heavy Metal Toxicity, Depression, Chronic Yeast Infection, Mycoplasma Infection, Obesity, Internal Alcoholism, Celiac Disease, Immune System Dysfunction, Enzyme Deficiency, Leaky Gut Syndrome and other maladies**, all which are revealed in this book.

This is the story of how Marc discovered with his doctors, healers and wife, the mysterious, underlying causes of his illnesses, and how he miraculously recovered his health over many decades using many unconventional methods to become an author, attorney, loving husband, caregiver, mentor, spiritual counselor, singer, world traveler, motorcyclist, and scuba diver.

During his recovery, he was co-chair of The Chronic Fatigue Syndrome and Fibromyalgia Research and Support Group of San Diego, California, with Ms. Jo Nost for more five years in the 1990's. The group had more than 400 members, most of whom had CFS and Fibromyalgia, but a few were their supporters and caregivers.

Marc's recovery is remarkable because his brain and most of his bodily systems were substantially impaired.

Along his "Road to Recovery," Marc made some amazing personal and medical discoveries, while answering some very basic questions, which had gone unanswered by his primary doctors for over 17 years:

(1) Why am I ill?

(2) What can I do about it?

He wrote this book because he wants to help the people who suffer from the same illnesses he did.

He wants them to receive the kind of care or better from their doctors, dentists, healers, medical consultants, caregivers, family, friends and support system that he did on his "Road to Recovery."

Simply put, he wants them to have the information that helped him recover from his illnesses, but faster, and with less pain and suffering.

61

Silver Linings

There were a few good things that came about because of Marc's illnesses and his "Road to Recovery."

First, Because of Marc's knowledge he gathered on his "Road to Recovery," he was able to give some people hope and a plan of action in their time of despair. For some, he was able to help them overcome their urge to commit suicide; get them to seek help from appropriate medical sources; and help them go on to live better, happier lives and enjoy major recoveries. He is very humbled and blessed for that honor.

Second, when Marc and his wife were visiting Israel in 1994, they saw that the Israelis were still using leaded gasoline. From his own personal struggle to overcome the toxic effects of lead poisoning, he understood quite clearly that kind of damage the Israeli's were inflicting upon their children.

On his return to the U.S., he wrote the Israeli leaders, reminding them of the dangers leaded gasoline posed to their children's health. Within a month, Israel began phasing out the use of leaded gasoline. Thank God for that one.

Third, during his recovery process, Marc came to understand that good food is required for recovery and healthy living. One day, he was visiting a dear friend who was recovering in a hospital in Ohio. He saw that the hospital was feeding his friend very unhealthy food.

On his return to San Diego, Marc wrote the hospital's directors and expressed his concerns. Once they realized that they could serve better quality food at no additional cost, they changed their ways. Again, Marc felt fortunate to have been a catalyst for constructive change.

If Marc had not become ill and had been forced by his life's circumstances to spend so much time and effort learning about how to recover from his many illnesses, he is certain that he would not have been able to help (1) a few people overcome their despair and recover, (2) Israel begin using unleaded gasoline; and (3) a teaching hospital provide healthier food to its patients.

It is obvious that those blessings were directly related to and caused by Marc's recovery process.

Tikkun Olam

62

For More Information

For additional books, e-books, and other products as they become available, please visit our website at:

www.RoadToRecoveryBook.com

Contact the author at:

RoadToRecoveryBook@gmail.com

63

Thank You
Very much for
Reading my book.

I wish you
Good luck,
Good health, and
Godspeed.

Marc Herlands, PWC

www.ingramcontent.com/pod-product-compliance
Lightning Source LLC
Chambersburg PA
CBHW080244290526
45790CB00005B/1690

* 9 7 8 1 4 8 1 9 1 6 9 1 2 *